THE INFLAMMATION DIET FOR BEGINNERS

100 Essential Anti-Inflammatory Diet Recipes

14 DAY MEAL PLAN   **20** FOODS TO AVOID   **10** WAYS TO REDUCE INFLAMMATION

TABLE OF CONTENTS

1

WHAT IS INFLAMMATION?

We live in a day and age when our food choices have significant impacts—on our health and well-being, the health and well-bring of those around us, and our environment. Modern food, adapted to our industrialized economy, is often radically different in nutritive value, appearance, and taste than the food our parents and grandparents ate. Even if you are a savvy shopper, it can be difficult to know exactly what you are putting into your body and how the foods you choose impact your overall health. Today, we are seeing diseases in startling numbers that, only a generation ago, were uncommon or rare. Perhaps not surprisingly, we now spend only 5 percent of our net income on food. A generation ago, it was 16 percent. Where did the other 11 percent go? Some of the money we used to spend on healthful food, we now spend on health care.

One condition that has risen to the top of the list of health concerns by medical practitioners as well as culinary consultants, dieticians, chefs, and others who work in the areas of food and health is inflammation. Inflammation is our body's protective biological response to harmful stimuli. In an effort to protect our system from a pathogen and to promote healing, our body launches an inflammation response.

These pathogens or invaders that promote an inflammatory response can be as seemingly innocuous as air pollution or dust, or as infections such as the common cold. Every day, we learn more about the dietary imbalances and deficiencies that often, at their root cause, are driven by our modern diets. This book seeks to provide you with information you can use to strengthen your body's response to inflammation and to reduce inflammation, by looking at our modern diet as a primary cause of inflammation. Foods with the nutrients that support our health can correct our dietary imbalances and reduce inflammation. Our diet can be the single most important tool in our tool kit to reduce inflammation and return our bodies to optimum health. As the old adage goes, "You are what you eat." Eat to reduce inflammation.

Signs and Symptoms of Inflammation

The onset of inflammation can be as silent as the growth of the trees outside your window. Most often, we experience inflammation as a daily inconvenience. Many of the ailments whose occurrences have risen exponentially during recent decades are attributed to inflammation, including allergies and food sensitivities, obesity and diabetes, asthma, arthritis, and cardiovascular disease.

Allergies and Food Sensitivities

In the United States there has been an 18 percent increase in environmental and food allergies over the last ten years. The most common allergic pollens are from grasses and weeds, such as ragweed, but many people are also sensitive to everyday mold and dust. When you inhale these allergens, the body's inflammation response causes tissue damage to the upper airway, causing you to sneeze or your nose to run.

Food sensitivities are also allergic responses, with symptoms that range from none at all to lactose intolerance, acne, eczema, osteoporosis, nausea, fatigue, itchy scalp, rashes, and a whole host of other symptoms. Modern wheat has recently come under fire as a trigger for inflammation (see page 12). Food sensitivities are more scientifically controversial because of the difficulty of identifying a reaction.

Food allergies can be life-threatening if your immune response is acute enough to obstruct airways, making breathing difficult or impossible. This is the case for some who are allergic to peanuts, shellfish, or strawberries, for example. The causes of food allergies are continually debated and range from an addiction to processed foods (which trigger euphoria) to celiac disease, where the immune response to gluten damages the intestinal wall.

Asthma

Asthma rates are on the rise, doubling throughout the 1990s and 2000s. Asthma is an inflammation response of the airways or passages of the lungs. The inflammatory response leads to the production of inflammatory messengers, and the airways, the bronchi and bronchioles, become swollen and inflamed. Breathing becomes difficult as the airway wall muscles begin to spasm.

Asthma can begin when the immune system becomes sensitized to an allergen, such as pet dander or pollen. Other factors that trigger asthmatic reactions include exercise, cold air, sulfites, and emotional stress.

Arthritis

Arthritis used to be considered a disease of old age, but in recent years more than 65 percent of arthritis has been diagnosed in people under the age of sixty-five. Perhaps not surprisingly, we are twice as likely to develop arthritis as our parents were. One in five Americans now suffers from arthritis.

- Osteoarthritis, the most common form of arthritis, is a progressive degenerative joint disease characterized by the breakdown of joint cartilage associated with risk factors such as obesity, history of joint injury, and age.
- Rheumatoid arthritis is the inflammation of the membranes lining the joint, which causes pain, stiffness, warmth, swelling, and sometimes severe joint damage.
- *Juvenile arthritis* is an umbrella term used to describe the many autoimmune and inflammatory conditions that can develop in children ages sixteen and younger.

The immune response attempts to repair damaged cells such as strained tendons. The wear and tear of daily life is certainly a factor, but the strain on your joints and the resulting inflammation is exacerbated by overuse and by carrying extra weight. As little as ten pounds of additional weight can have a tremendous impact on your body. Worse, injured tissues anywhere in the body—lungs, nose, intestine, joints— are more susceptible to repeated injury and to chronic inflammation.

Obesity and Diabetes

Diabetes is characterized by chronic elevated levels of blood sugar and insulin. Almost 20 million Americans suffer from diabetes, a 49 percent increase from a decade ago. The cause? Increased levels of glucose start a chain reaction that stimulates the inflammatory response. The constant inflammatory stimulation increases the diabetic's risk of developing other diseases such as blindness, heart disease, and cancer. Research into the causes of diabetes continues, but a growing body of scientists point to human evolution and its collision with modern dietary practices. Our bodies are simply not adapted to modern foods.

Nearly 36 percent of Americans are obese, thirty or more pounds over their ideal weight, a rate that has nearly tripled in sixteen years. How our bodies process a modern diet of high sugar and high carbohydrates triggers a stronger insulin response and serves to elevate glucose levels, which, through our body's natural processes, stimulates the inflammatory response. Recent research has demonstrated a previously unknown fact: our fat cells have a metabolic function. Historically, the inflammation response was helpful for our ancient ancestors, who ate a limited diet, to survive any number of infectious diseases. With obesity, a condition of abundance, the inflammation response from metabolically active fat cells is multiplied. Our overflowing food cornucopia, a benefit of our modern society, results in negative consequences.

Cardiovascular Disease

Coronary artery disease occurs when plaque builds up in the arteries that supply blood to the heart. Plaque is made up of cholesterol deposits, which can accumulate in your arteries. This plaque buildup effectively narrows the artery, causing your heart to work harder to move blood through the restricted arteries. This process is called atherosclerosis. It is estimated that over 60 million Americans have coronary artery disease.

Cholesterol is just one of many factors now believed to contribute to heart disease. Nutritional deficiencies and inflammatory injury to artery walls as a result of these nutritional deficiencies are as impactful as cholesterol on heart health. To understand this a bit more, let's look at the amino acid homocysteine.

Elevated homocysteine levels in the blood can damage the lining of the arteries and may make blood clot more easily than it should, resulting in an increase in the risk of blood vessel blockages. Most people who have a high homocysteine level do not get enough folate (also called folic acid), vitamin B_6, or vitamin B_{12} in their diet. Restoring these vitamins by eating foods that contain these nutrients helps return homocysteine levels to normal. Further research has demonstrated that modest supplements of folic acid, vitamin B_6, and vitamin B_{12} inhibited the inflammation process in blood vessel walls and significantly lowered homocysteine levels.

The role of inflammation in cardiovascular disease has become even more comprehensively understood, in part because of the widespread availability of a test for C–reactive protein (CRP) levels. The CRP test, now a common test for inflammation, looks at your CRP, as found in arterial lesions. Not all lesions contain CRP, but those that do are unstable and likely to lead to breakaway fragments and clots. Formerly seen as a marker of the body's inflammatory response postinjury, CRP at higher levels in the blood is known to indicate high plaque production levels. A high CRP reading is considered a more reliable predictor of heart disease than either high cholesterol or high homocysteine levels.

2

INFLAMMATION AND DIET

The primary causes of inflammation are often related to dietary imbalances or nutritional deficiencies. When reducing inflammation it is important to identify and reduce the causes of inflammation. By avoiding specific foods you are allergic to or limiting your exposure to airborne toxins that could result in an asthma attack, you can reduce the agitation of your immune system.

Environmental stresses such as tobacco smoke and air pollution irritate the lungs and can trigger the immune response, as can environmental allergies to pollen, dust, and mold. Food allergies and sensitivities can cause allergic or allergic-like reactions that trigger the immune response.

We have already discussed some of the problems caused by our modern diet's reliance on refined carbohydrates and sugar. Another dietary imbalance that promotes inflammation is consuming too many fats.

The Importance of Fats

All humans need fats in their diets for optimum health. But to reduce inflammation, we must review the types of fats we are eating and look at how much of each type of fat we consume in relation to other fats. The human body metabolizes fat just as it always has, but modern diets include types and amounts of fats that the body is not prepared to handle. Here is a closer look at these fats and what happens when we eat them.

Omega-6

Called an "essential" fat because our body cannot produce it on its own, Omega-6 is in just about everything we eat that contains fat, including meat, dairy, and eggs. Vegetable oils, such as corn oil, soybean oil, sunflower oil, and safflower oil, are good sources for Omega-6. Soybean oil and corn oil are in just about every packaged food on the shelf; flip over a bottle of your favorite bottled salad dressing, and you are likely to see soybean or corn oil as the first ingredient. Now examine a package of bread or crackers, or a soda can, or countless other packaged goods. These oils, by-products of our modern industrial agricultural system, are ubiquitous. While some amount of Omega-6 is necessary, all that extra Omega-6 is sending shockwaves through our bodies as inflammation.

The mechanism behind inflammation is the process by which our bodies synthesize Omega-6, or linoleic acid (LA). When we digest LA, our body, through a series of chemical processes, changes LA into another fatty acid called gammalinolenic acid (GLA) and subsequently produces an inflammatory messenger called arachidonic acid (AA). Luckily for us, our bodies are not very good at converting LA into GLA, so our production of inflammatory messengers is limited. But most of us eating a modern diet have high levels of AA in our blood.

Omega-3

Another essential fatty acid, Omega-3, is known to reduce triglycerides, high amounts of which are an important predictor of heart disease. Just as with Omega-6, our bodies do not naturally produce Omega-3, so we must consume it in our food to benefit from its healing properties. Omega-3 is found in vegetarian foods such as flaxseeds and chia seeds, oils, eggs, and fatty fish such as salmon. The fatty acids that result from metabolizing Omega-3 from plants are known as alpha-linolenic acid or ALA. Omega-3 metabolized from fish, such as cod liver, herring, mackerel, salmon, or sardines, is called eicosapentaenoic acid (EPA) and docosahexaenoic acid (DHA). DHA can also be synthesized from ALA.

Omega-6 and Omega-3 Together

In tandem, Omega-6 and Omega-3 reduce our risk of heart, brain, and liver disorders, sterility, susceptibility to infections, vision impairment, and learning disabilities. However, not all Omega-6s are created equal. The "good" Omega-6 is the one that helps our bodies block the conversion of AA into inflammatory messengers; this Omega-6 is known as dihomogammalinolenic acid (DGLA). DGLA is not readily available in our food supply, so we must eat something that our body can convert into DGLA. That something is gammalinolenic acid, the GLA mentioned earlier. GLA is naturally occurring in black currant oil, pine nuts, evening primrose oil, and borage seed oil.

A note of caution, however: adding too much GLA to our bodies without the counterbalance of a certain type of Omega-3 has negative effects. Excess GLA moves to the liver, where it is converted to AA. Fortunately, this effect can be blocked by increasing our consumption of EPA, the Omega-3 long-chain fatty acid known as eicosapentaenoic acid. It turns out that our grandparents were onto something when they took their spoonful of cod liver oil every day—it is rich in those balancing EPAs.

A study published in the *New England Journal of Medicine* in 2002 demonstrated the link between AA and heart disease; a genetic predisposition to heart disease is tied to the way AA is processed. The study also found that atherosclerosis and related heart disease were worse in patients who ate a diet that contained high levels of AA.

To reduce inflammation and prevent new inflammation, the balance of Omega-6 as DGLA to Omega-3 as EPA turns out to be the critical piece of the puzzle.

Omega-9

Omega-9, or monounsaturated oleic and stearic acid, is a nonessential fatty acid produced naturally by the body whenever there is enough of either Omega-6 or Omega-3. Omega-9 is found in olives, avocados, macadamia nuts, pistachios, pecans, and other nuts. By improving your Omega-3 and Omega-6 levels, you will naturally increase your Omega-9 levels.

Fish

Doctors now recommend that we eat more fish, an important source of essential fatty acids. But in response to overfishing, as well as the declining health of oceans and freshwater streams where fatty fish spend most of their lives, fish, too, have become a modern agricultural product; increasingly, the fish that we buy in the supermarket is farm-raised.

Farmed salmon eat what the farmer provides for them, which is often feed such as soy, corn, and wheat, which can result in high levels of AA, the very opposite of what most of us have heard about the fatty acid benefits of salmon.

Wild salmon, on the other hand, eat algae primarily. Algae are rich in Omega-3 fatty acids, and wild salmon easily convert their dietary Omega-3s to EPA and DHA.

Eggs

Eggs have been a controversial food for so long, many of us avoid eating them. To reduce inflammation, the egg's nutritional aspects must be considered. The yolk contains high amounts of cholesterol and significant amounts of AA. Even eggs from chickens fed Omega-3s as part of their diet to boost an egg's Omega-3 levels still contain the same amount of AA per yolk (about 141 milligrams) as those fed a regular diet. However, egg whites and egg substitutes, made primarily of egg whites, do not contain AA.

Back to Balance

Reducing the overall amount of AA in your system is an important step in reducing inflammation. Since many modern foods rely heavily on oils and other products with Omega-6 fats, and we are eating many more refined carbohydrates and sugar than ever before, our diets are no longer in balance for optimal health.

As we know from our ancestors, humans historically needed a certain amount of Omega-6 and its resulting AA to fight off any number of infections. Until about eighty years ago, Americans ate a 2:1 ratio of Omega-6 to Omega-3 fats. The ratio of Omega-6 to Omega-3 in our diets today is closer to 20:1. We now consume too many Omega-6 fatty acids and not enough Omega-3.

Trans-Fats and Saturated vs. Unsaturated Fats

All of the fatty acids discussed earlier are unsaturated fats. Omega-6 and Omega-3 are polyunsaturated fats. Both polyunsaturated and monounsaturated fats may help lower your blood cholesterol level when you use them in place of saturated fats and trans-fats. Saturated fats come mostly from animal products and do not lower cholesterol.

Trans-fatty acids (TFA) are found in small amounts in various animal products such as beef, pork, lamb, and the butterfat in butter and milk. TFA are also formed during the process of hydrogenation, making margarine, shortening, cooking oils, and the foods made from them a major source of TFA in the American diet.

Modern Wheat

In the years since World War II, wheat has gone through a massive transformation. The goal during the war was to increase wheat yields globally and thus reduce hunger by breeding wheat strains that could be easily and efficiently threshed, the process of separating the edible grain from the inedible chaff. Years of hybridization have resulted in the development of thousands of new strains of wheat. The most high-yielding of these have been adopted worldwide, which has gone a long way to reducing world hunger. But there is a catch, of course.

The new dwarf and semi-dwarf wheat, with short stalks to ease the threshing process, now comprise more than 99 percent of all wheat grown worldwide. After these countless hybridizations, *Triticum aestivum*, or common wheat, is structurally different than ancient or unhybridized forms of wheat. Common wheat expresses a higher quantity of genes for wheat-gluten proteins. Not only are there structural changes in the proteins but also there are new proteins that were not part of the parent plant's gene structure. There is a significant health issue related to modern wheat and its impact on blood sugar.

The Glycemic Index and High-Glycemic Foods

Gram for gram, wheat increases blood sugar to a greater degree than other carbohydrates, such as chickpeas or even potato chips. This has to do with the carbohydrate structure of these foods and how our digestive system converts the carbohydrates in wheat to glucose. The carbohydrates in wheat are 75 percent amylopectin A and 25 percent amylose. Our bodies easily digest the amylopectin A and rapidly convert it to glucose. (Amylose is much less efficiently digested.)

A comparative look at the blood sugar impacts of carbohydrates was done as long ago as 1981, when a study at the University of Toronto launched the concept of the glycemic index (GI). Specifically, the higher the blood sugar after consuming a specific food compared to glucose, the higher the GI. In that study, the GI of white bread was 69, while the GI of whole-grain bread was 72. Sucrose (table sugar) was 59. At the root, it is the body's ease of digesting the amylopectin A that gives wheat bread and white bread a GI higher than table sugar.

This book does not suggest that you completely eliminate wheat from your diet. However, to reduce inflammation, the type of wheat you choose can have a significant impact on your health. Ancient, pre-hybridized forms of wheat still contain gluten, and some can have a higher glycemic load. But this book will propose alternatives to modern wheat.

3

REDUCING INFLAMMATION

A Return to Heritage Foods

Human bodies have not changed much in the past 50,000 or so years, but dramatic changes to the foods we eat—which ones and in what quantities—are having a profound impact on our health and the health of our environment. When you decrease the modern, heavily processed foods you consume and increase the traditional foods you eat, your risk of inflammation and the problems, consequences, and diseases associated with inflammation can be reduced.

We live in a time of tremendous choice in what we are able to eat, but from this huge, sometimes overwhelming spectrum, a small shift in what we eat can have profound consequences on our health.

To reduce inflammation and get our bodies back into balance, a diet should reduce these items:

> ➢ Trans-fats and saturated fats
> ➢ Soy, corn, and sunflower oils

> Conventionally grown fruits and vegetables (pesticide residues on conventionally grown crops may trigger the inflammatory response)
> Beverages with sugar or sugar substitutes
> Carbohydrates that are high glycemic
> Egg yolk
> Farmed salmon and other farmed fish
> Processed foods, especially carbohydrates
> High-gluten wheat (modern, conventional wheat)

And increase these items:

> Organic fruits and vegetables
> Wild salmon and other wild fatty fish
> Nuts and seeds such as walnuts, pistachios, pine nuts, and cashews
> Olive, walnut, and canola oil
> Egg whites
> Lower-gluten whole grains such as spelt, barley, and rye, and no-gluten whole grains such as quinoa and millet
> Whole foods that are minimally processed

Some Questions—and Answers—about Eating to Reduce Inflammation

What is the optimum amount of fish to eat to reduce inflammation?

A small portion of fatty wild fish such as anchovies, herring, mackerel, and wild Alaskan salmon every day can significantly contribute to the amount of eicosapentaenoic acid (EPA) in your blood.

I've heard that I should limit the amount of fish I eat because so many fish are contaminated with mercury. If farmed salmon is not safe (from an arachidonic acid [AA] perspective), is wild salmon safe from a mercury perspective?

In a 2008 study published in *Environmental Toxicology and Chemistry*, wild Canadian salmon was found to have mercury levels three times higher than farmed. However, mercury levels in both farmed and wild Canadian salmon (the kinds most consumed in the United States) were significantly below human health guidelines.

As a vegetarian I do not eat fish and would prefer not to take supplements containing fish by-products. Are there any alternatives for me to get the EPA and docosahexaenoic acid (DHA) I need?

A series of new investigations into plant seeds that contain a fatty acid called stearidonic acid is underway. Stearidonic acid appears to have similar biological properties to EPA and could one day be an alternative to fish oil. However, as of this writing, no vegetarian supplement exists that can entirely replicate the beneficial anti-inflammatory effects of fish oil. Camelina oil and chia seeds, two newer products on the market, offer high levels of Omega-3, but studies have not yet confirmed the body's ability to metabolize camelina oil. Echium oil is another new oil entering the market that has high levels of stearidonic acid.

Flaxseeds have been touted as a vegetarian alternative, but it turns out we do not easily convert the fatty acid in flaxseeds (LNA) into EPA and DHA. While better than consuming soybean oil, flaxseeds do not carry the same anti-inflammatory benefits as eating EPA and DHA from wild salmon.

I am concerned about eating fish for environmental reasons. Are there fish that are good choices for me to eat?

Alaskan salmon, including wild Chinook and sockeye, are "best choices" on the most current Monterey Bay Aquarium's Seafood Watch list. Other fatty fish, such as anchovies and herring, are also "best choices" and, because of their small size and relatively short life compared to big fish like salmon and halibut, have minimal mercury risk. Pacific halibut, a "best choice" from an environmental perspective, is not a good choice from an inflammation perspective, as it contains higher AA levels. Farmed Atlantic salmon is to be avoided from both perspectives.

Legumes are high on the glycemic index. Why are they included here?

Amylopectin C, the glucose derived from legumes, is the least digestible carbohydrate. Undigested amylopectin C moves through your digestive system without being converted to sugar.

Hemp seeds are high in Omega-3 fat. Do I need to eat the seeds to get the nutritional benefits, or is hemp milk an acceptable substitute?

You do not need to eat hemp seeds. Both hemp milk and hemp oil provide the benefits of Omega-3.

10 Tips to Achieve Lasting Change

1. Finding balance is the key to success. Choose foods and meals that offer a balance of protein, fat, and carbohydrates.
2. Choose foods that are high in antioxidants, such as leafy greens and berries. Think of a prism or rainbow and all of the colors contained in a rainbow. Eat fruits and vegetables that are colorful and come from all colors of the rainbow.
3. Fattier cuts of meat such as pepperoni, sausage, bacon, or beef stew are fine in moderation. Aim to reduce these foods in your diet to a few times a week and increase consumption of lower-fat meats and heart-healthful fats.
4. An important source of calcium, whole-fat dairy helps us feel full. When shopping, read ingredient labels and select dairy products where the first ingredient is milk.
5. Planning meals and snacks in advance reduces the likelihood of overeating at snack and meal times.
6. When dining out, research the restaurant beforehand to confirm that they can offer you a meal that works with your dietary needs.

Most restaurants will happily accommodate requests if they are provided in advance of the meal.

7. It can take some time for our palates to adjust to a new diet. Small changes can have a big impact. As a starting point, select one food you enjoy eating and look for similar foods that are less inflammatory. Once the new food has been incorporated into your diet, take steps to make other small changes. The Meatless Monday initiative, begun a few years ago, is a simple way to rethink what and how you eat. Instead of eating meat on Monday, replace the meat you would have eaten with fish or vegetables. Voilà, you have changed 15 percent of your meals in favor of your health.

8. Try not to think of foods you "cannot" or "should not" eat. The goal is not to eliminate your favorite foods but to shift the balance of the foods you eat to reduce or prevent inflammation.

9. Put fish on the menu at least three times a week.

10. Choose carbohydrates carefully. Look for carbohydrates that have at least 5 grams of dietary fiber per serving. For optimal satiety, also look for foods that have 4 grams of protein per serving. Increase fiber slowly. Your digestive tract needs time to adjust to any changes.

Anti-Inflammatory Foods

The following list shows what kinds of foods to include in your daily diet. Keep in mind, though, that with so many healing foods to choose from, these choices are a guideline to help you get started.

- Fish, including anchovies, herring, mackerel, sardines, trout, and wild Alaskan salmon
- Shellfish, including crab, mussels, oysters, and shrimp
- Seaweed and sea vegetables, such as dulse and nori
- Lean meats and poultry, including buffalo, leaner cuts of grass-fed beef, lamb, pork, chicken, and turkey

- Plant-based oils, such as olive, canola, flaxseeds, and coconut
- Whole-milk dairy and cheese
- Egg whites
- Beans and legumes, such as chickpeas, lentils, and split peas
- Organic soybeans in the form of tofu or whole beans (edamame)
- Nuts, such as almonds, walnuts, and hazelnuts. Enjoy these whole or as milks and oils, too.
- Seeds, such as chia, hemp, flax, sesame. Enjoy these whole or as milks and oils, too.
- Gluten-free whole grains that are minimally processed, such as quinoa, buckwheat, oats, and brown rice
- Heritage varieties of gluten-bearing, minimally processed grains, such as farro, spelt, and rye
- Vegetables (organic whenever possible), including celery, cucumbers, green beans and root vegetables (turnip, parsnip, rutabaga), squash, sweet potato and carrots. All of the dark green, leafy vegetables (kale, cabbage, turnip greens, collard greens, broccoli, cauliflower) are also high in phytonutrients and soluble fiber.
- Fruits (organic whenever possible), including apples, avocados, berries (strawberry, blueberry, blackberry), stone fruits (cherry, peach, plum, apricot), figs, pears, limes, and lemons
- Dark chocolate

Inflammatory Foods to Avoid

Some foods promote inflammation and these should be avoided.

- Any food containing artificial color, flavor, or other chemical ingredients
- Artificial sweeteners, such as aspartame and saccharin
- Monosodium glutamate (MSG)
- Beverages with sugar or sugar substitutes
- Soybean, corn, sunflower, and safflower oils

- High-gluten wheat (modern, conventional wheat), including commercial baked goods, crackers, and bread
- Foods made from white or whole-wheat flour, including commercial baked goods, crackers, and white bread
- Instant rice
- Instant oatmeal
- Conventionally grown fruits and vegetables (pesticide residues on conventionally grown crops may trigger the inflammatory response)
- White potatoes, including French fries
- Processed and fried vegetables, such as onion rings and potato chips
- Canned fruit preserved in corn syrup or sugar
- Egg yolks
- Farmed salmon, halibut, and other farmed fish
- Deli meats
- Organ meats

4

14-DAY MEAL PLAN

To help get you started on the path to good health, here are two weeks' worth of menus. Recipes for all the dishes are included in this book.

Week One

Vegetarian Monday

Breakfast: Hot Quinoa Breakfast Cereal with Fruit and Flaxseeds (page 66)
Lunch: Open-Faced Eggplant Parmesan Sandwiches (page 33)
Snack: Classic Hummus (page 73)
Dinner: Yellow Dal with Split Peas (page 77)

Low-Carb/Low-Gluten Tuesday

Breakfast: Fresh Veggie Frittata (page 126)
Lunch: Coleslaw Chicken Salad with Asian Flavors (page 117)
Snack: Dark-Chocolate Nut Clusters (page 131)
Dinner: Lamb Kebabs with Garlic and Mint (page 111)

Midweek Treat

Breakfast: Banana-Blueberry Muffins (page 60)
Lunch: Salmon Poke (page 87)
Snack: Chocolate Pudding (page 132)
Dinner: Turkey-Spinach Meatloaf (page 118)

Colorful Thursday

Breakfast: Peachy Green Smoothie (page 45)
Lunch: Mediterranean Tuna Salad Sandwiches (page 93)
Snack: Baked Kale Chips (page 27)
Dinner: Black-Eyed-Pea Burgers (page 79)

Friday Means Fish

Breakfast: Salmon Scramble Sandwich (page 129)
Lunch: Herring with Mustard and Dill Salad (page 99)
Snack: Versatile Cracker Spread (page 121)
Dinner: Trout and Parma Ham (page 96)

Weekend Slowdown

Saturday

Breakfast: Pumpkin Polenta Pancakes (page 25)
Lunch: Warm Spinach and Mushroom Salad (page 30)
Snack: Cornmeal Halva (page 72)
Dinner: Cioppino (page 105)

Sunday

Breakfast: Breakfast Rice (page 61)
Lunch: Dolmas Wraps (page 64)
Snack: Coconut Date Bars (page 53)
Dinner: Grilled Skirt Steak with Salsa Verde (page 107)

Week Two

Vegetarian Monday
Breakfast: Hazelnut-Banana Open-Faced Sandwiches (page 84)
Lunch: Cold Soba Noodles with Peanut Sauce (page 70)
Snack: Almond-Honey Power Bars (page 82)
Dinner: Spiced Sweet Potatoes with Peas and Cauliflower (page 41)

Low-Carb/Low-Gluten Tuesday
Breakfast: Plantains with Greek Yogurt and Honey (page 46)
Lunch: Swiss Chard with White Beans and Bell Peppers (page 40)
Snack: Fresh Figs with Chocolate Sauce (page 55)
Dinner: Pork Chops with Double Pumpkin (page 115)

Midweek Treat
Breakfast: Flaxseed and Cranberry Muffins (page 58)
Lunch: Egg Drop Soup (page 127)
Snack: Roasted Mixed Nuts with Tamari (page 81)
Dinner: Grilled Herbed Tuna (page 94)

Colorful Thursday
Breakfast: Pears with Blue Cheese and Walnuts (page 50)
Lunch: Tabbouleh (page 65)
Snack: Cocoa and Coconut Banana Slices (page 54)
Dinner: Mackerel and Lentil Salad (page 100)

Friday Means Fish
Breakfast: Fish Tacos (page 95)
Lunch: Shrimp Soup with Leeks and Fennel (page 102)
Snack: Chili Shrimp (page 103)
Dinner: Mussels in Tomato Sugo (page 104)

Weekend Slowdown

Saturday

    Breakfast: Cornmeal Baklava (page 85)
    Lunch: Farro Bean Soup (page 69)
    Snack: Honeydew Melon and Berries (page 47)
    Dinner: Smoky Buffalo Burgers (page 112)

Sunday

    Breakfast: Apple, Peach, and Acorn Squash "Pie" (page 51)
    Lunch: Fennel and Celery Salad with Dates (page 29)
    Snack: Marinated Olives and Mushrooms (page 28)
    Dinner: Mustard-Crusted Salmon (page 91)

5

VEGETABLES

Pumpkin Polenta Pancakes

Makes 8–1o Pancakes

It sounds like breakfast but the savory combination of pumpkin, polenta, and kefir makes this a great appetizer or snack. You can use agave nectar instead of maple syrup for a more neutral flavor.

For the pancakes:

- 2 cups water
- Pinch of salt
- 1½ cups cornmeal
- Sea salt and freshly ground black pepper
- 6 tablespoons olive oil
- 5-pound baking pumpkin, such as Amish paste, peeled, seeded, and cut into 1-inch chunks (about 2 cups)
- ¼ cup maple syrup
- 1 tablespoon grape-seed oil

For the sauce:

- 1 cup kefir
- 1 tablespoon honey
- ½ cup toasted walnuts, chopped
- Fresh mint and star fruit, for garnish

---

continued ▶

Pumpkin Polenta Pancake *continued* ▶

Preheat the oven to 375°F.

To make the pancakes:
1. Bring water and a pinch of salt to a boil in a medium saucepan over high heat. Slowly add 1 cup of the cornmeal, stirring constantly with a wooden spoon for 7 to 10 minutes. Reduce the heat to medium. Before the polenta starts to thicken, season with sea salt and pepper and add 2 tablespoons off the olive oil. Stir until thick. Remove from the heat and let cool.

2. In the meantime, place the pumpkin on a greased baking pan, drizzle with maple syrup and grape-seed oil, and bake in the oven for 15 to 20 minutes until golden brown. Remove from the oven, allow to cool, and place in a large bowl. Mash pumpkin with a potato masher.

3. Add the cooked polenta to the bowl with the pumpkin and stir to combine. Shape the mixture into patties.

4. Place the remaining ½ cup cornmeal in a shallow dish such as a pie pan. Coat each pumpkin patty with cornmeal. Heat a nonstick sauté pan with the remaining 4 tablespoons olive oil until shimmering. Fry pumpkin patties until both sides are golden brown, about 4 minutes per side.

To make the sauce:
Mix the kefir, honey, and walnuts in a bowl. Place the pumpkin polenta pancakes onto plates and pour sauce over top. Garnish with mint and star fruit and serve.

Baked Kale Chips

Makes About 4 Cups

If you're looking for a crunchy snack to munch on instead of potato chips, you'll love these kale chips. Kale is extremely low in calories and is one of the most nutrient-dense foods on the planet. Crunchy and flavorful, these chips will help you meet your daily requirement of vegetables.

- 2 heads curly leaf kale
- 2 tablespoons olive oil
- Sea salt

---

1. Preheat the oven to 325°F. Tear the kale into bite-size pieces, removing any tough stems, and place in a medium bowl. Add the olive oil.

2. Using your hands, massage the olive oil into the kale, and then lay the kale on a baking sheet in a single layer. Sprinkle with sea salt.

3. Bake for 10 to 15 minutes until crispy. Serve or store in an airtight container.

Marinated Olives and Mushrooms

Makes 8 Servings

Tangy and salty olives combine with mild button mushrooms to make a marinated treat. These savory morsels are easy to prepare and are especially good to serve at a party. Store in the refrigerator for up to 3 days, but serve at room temperature.

- 1 pound white button mushrooms
- 1 pound mixed, high-quality olives
- 2 tablespoons fresh thyme leaves
- 1 tablespoon white wine vinegar
- ½ tablespoon crushed fennel seeds
- Pinch of chili flakes
- Olive oil, to cover
- Sea salt and freshly ground black pepper

1. Clean and rinse mushrooms under cold water and pat dry.

2. Combine mushrooms, olives, thyme, white wine vinegar, fennel seeds, and chili flakes in a glass jar or other airtight container. Cover with olive oil and season with sea salt and freshly ground pepper. Shake to distribute the ingredients.

3. Allow to marinate for at least 1 hour. Serve at room temperature.

Fennel and Celery Salad with Dates

Makes 6 Servings

Your taste buds will rejoice with this salad's medley of flavors. Sweet dates and fennel, sour lemon, bitter celery, and salty cheese combine to make this a crowd pleaser.

- ½ cup toasted almonds, coarsely chopped
- 8 celery stalks, cut on the diagonal into ½-inch slices, leaves reserved
- ½ fennel bulb, cut into ½-inch slices, stalks discarded, fronds reserved
- 6 dates, pitted and coarsely chopped
- 3 tablespoons fresh lemon juice
- Sea salt and freshly ground black pepper
- 2 ounces Grana Padano, shaved
- ¼ cup olive oil
- Crushed red pepper flakes

Toss the almonds, celery, celery leaves, fennel, dates, and lemon juice in a medium bowl; season with salt and pepper. Add the Grana Padano and oil and toss gently; sprinkle the red pepper flakes on top and garnish with the reserved fennel fronds.

Warm Spinach and Mushroom Salad

Makes 2 Servings

A bit of bacon adds oomph to this winter salad. In spring, add a few fresh artichoke hearts.

- 5 tablespoons olive oil
- ¼ cup diced pancetta
- ½ cup sliced button mushrooms
- ½ teaspoon dried thyme
- ½ small red onion, thinly sliced
- 2 cups baby spinach leaves

- ½ cup alfalfa sprouts
- 1 tomato, chopped
- ½ small cucumber, seeded and chopped
- Juice of 1 lemon
- Sea salt and freshly ground black pepper

---

1. In a medium nonstick skillet over medium-high heat, warm 3 tablespoons of the olive oil until shimmering. Add the pancetta, mushrooms, and thyme and cook, stirring occasionally, until the mushrooms begin to caramelize, about 5 minutes. Add the onion and cook just enough to soften, about 1 minute. Remove from the heat.

2. Meanwhile, place the spinach in a large salad bowl. Spoon the mushroom mix on top of greens. Toss to combine. Combine the sprouts, tomato, cucumber, remaining 2 tablespoons olive oil, and the lemon juice in a bowl, and season with sea salt and freshly ground pepper.

3. Toss the salad until well mixed and serve.

Carrot Coconut Salad

Makes 3–4 Servings

This salad gets a nutritional update with honey, coconut, and roasted pecans. Coconut oil and other whole coconut products are a good source of lauric acid, a saturated fatty acid that enhances the immune system.

- 2 tablespoons honey
- ½ teaspoon sea salt
- ¼ cup freshly squeezed orange juice
- 1 teaspoon freshly grated ginger
- 1 tablespoon coconut oil, softened
- 2 cups grated or julienned carrots
- 1 cup unsweetened coconut flakes
- ½ cup toasted, chopped pecans or cashews

In a medium bowl, mix the honey, sea salt, orange juice, ginger, and coconut oil. Mix in the carrots, coconut flakes, and pecans or cashews until the dressing evenly coats the salad. Serve.

Tomato Soup

Makes 6 Servings

This version of tomato soup is subtly flavored with the classic spices of Morocco—paprika, ginger, cumin, and cinnamon. In terms of nutrients, cooked tomatoes are a great source of lycopene.

- 2 tablespoons olive oil
- 1 large onion, coarsely chopped
- 8 large tomatoes, seeded and coarsely chopped
- 1 teaspoon paprika
- 1 teaspoon fresh ginger, finely chopped
- 1 teaspoon ground cumin
- 2 cups chicken broth
- 1 cinnamon stick
- 1 teaspoon honey
- Sea salt and freshly ground black pepper
- Juice of 1 lemon
- 1 small bunch flat-leaf parsley, chopped, for garnish
- 2 tablespoons chopped fresh cilantro, for garnish

1. Heat a large Dutch oven over medium-high heat. Add the olive oil and onion, and cook until soft and translucent. Add the tomatoes, paprika, ginger, and cumin and stir.

2. Pour in the chicken broth and add the cinnamon stick and honey. Simmer for 15 minutes. Purée the soup in a food processor or blender. (Remove the cinnamon stick for this step and return it to the pot when done.)

3. Pour the soup back into the pot and season with sea salt and freshly ground pepper. Stir in the lemon juice and serve garnished with the parsley and cilantro.

Open-Faced Eggplant Parmesan Sandwiches

Makes 1 Serving

Eggplant Parmesan is often deep-fried, laden with high-fat cheese, and served atop mounds of pasta. In this version, the eggplant is broiled before being topped with marinara and low-fat Parmesan cheese and served on a slice of toasted whole-grain bread. Eat with a knife and fork and enjoy!

- 1 small eggplant, sliced into ¼-inch rounds
- Pinch of sea salt
- 2 tablespoons olive oil
- Sea salt and freshly ground black pepper
- 2 slices quinoa, millet, or spelt bread, thickly cut and toasted
- 1 cup unsweetened marinara sauce, warmed
- ¼ cup freshly grated Parmesan cheese

1. Preheat the broiler to high.

2. Salt both sides of the sliced eggplant and let sit for 20 minutes.

3. Rinse the eggplant and pat dry with a paper towel. Brush the eggplant with the olive oil, and season with sea salt and freshly ground pepper.

4. Lay the eggplant on a sheet pan, and broil until crisp, about 4 minutes. Flip over and broil the other side, about 2 minutes.

5. Lay the toasted bread on a sheet pan. Spoon some marinara sauce on each slice of bread and layer the eggplant on top. Sprinkle half of the cheese on top of the eggplant and top with more marinara sauce. Sprinkle remaining cheese over the sauce, and serve immediately.

Green Beans with Peaches and Almonds

Makes 4 Servings

This is a summery update to the classic green bean almandine. In the fall, swap the peaches for plums or apples.

- 4 quarts water
- 1 pound trimmed green beans
- 2 peaches, cut into ½-inch wedges
- 2 tablespoons olive oil, plus more as needed
- 1 tablespoon fresh lemon juice
- ½ cup toasted almond slivers

1. Bring the water to a boil. Place the green beans in a steamer basket and steam 4 minutes until crisp-tender. Set aside.

2. Meanwhile, toss the peaches with the olive oil. Heat a grill pan or a sauté pan over medium-high heat and add the peaches, turning often, until they are lightly charred, about 8 minutes.

3. Add the green beans to the pan and a bit more olive oil if needed, and cook an additional 2 minutes. Remove from the heat. Toss with the lemon juice and toasted almonds, and serve.

Caramelized Root Vegetables

Makes 6 Servings

Slowly cooking the vegetables in this recipe will allow them to develop color and sweetness without burning. Don't skip the seasonings—spices have nutrients and antioxidant power.

- 2 medium carrots, peeled and cut into chunks
- 2 medium red or gold beets, peeled and cut into chunks
- 2 turnips, peeled and cut into chunks
- 2 tablespoons olive oil
- 1 teaspoon ground cumin
- 1 teaspoon sweet paprika
- Sea salt and freshly ground black pepper
- Juice of 1 lemon
- 1 small bunch flat-leaf parsley, chopped

---

1. Preheat the oven to 400°F.

2. Toss the vegetables with the olive oil, cumin, and paprika. Place in a single layer on a sheet pan, season with sea salt and freshly ground pepper, drizzle with lemon juice, and roast for 30 to 40 minutes, turning once, until veggies are slightly browned and crisp.

3. Serve warm, topped with the chopped parsley.

Roasted Beets with Orange Essence

Makes 6–8 Servings

For optimal flavor, look for fresh bunches of beets, with firm, unblemished skin and bright green tops.

- 2 pounds red beets, scrubbed clean, green tops removed and reserved for another use
- 3 tablespoons olive oil
- Sea salt
- ½ cup balsamic vinegar
- 2 teaspoons sugar (optional)
- 1 teaspoon grated orange zest
- Freshly ground black pepper

1. Preheat the oven to 400°F. Line a roasting pan with aluminum foil. Peel the beets and cut into quarters. Place the beets in the pan. Rub 1 tablespoon of the olive oil over the beets and sprinkle with salt. Cover the beets with another sheet of aluminum foil. Roast for 45 minutes to an hour, testing doneness by poking a beet with the tines of a fork. Once the fork tines go in easily, the beets are tender and cooked. Remove from the oven.

2. Toss the beets with the remaining 2 tablespoons olive oil, the vinegar, sugar, orange zest, and black pepper. Serve warm or cold.

Roasted Balsamic Brussels Sprouts with Pecans

Makes 4 Servings

This is a terrific recipe for those who say they don't like Brussels sprouts, as roasting them brings out their sweetness and the vinegar adds a refreshing tartness. Substitute walnuts or almonds for the pecans, if you prefer.

- 20 to 25 medium Brussels sprouts (about 1 pound), quartered
- 2 tablespoons olive oil
- 1 tablespoon balsamic vinegar
- Sea salt and freshly ground black pepper
- ¼ cup chopped pecans, toasted

1. Preheat the oven to 400°F.

2. Spread the Brussels sprouts on a single layer on a baking sheet. Drizzle with olive oil and vinegar, and sprinkle with sea salt and freshly ground pepper. Roast for 15 to 20 minutes, until tender and caramelized.

3. Top with the toasted pecans and serve.

Rosemary-Roasted Acorn Squash

Makes 4 Servings

When roasted at high heat, the skin of acorn squash becomes soft, tender, and edible. Meanwhile, the benefits of rosemary are many: it is thought to stimulate the immune system, increase circulation, and improve digestion.

- 1 acorn squash
- 2 tablespoons honey
- 2 tablespoons rosemary, finely chopped
- 2 tablespoons olive oil
- Sea salt

1. Preheat the oven to 400°F.

2. Cut the squash in half and scrape out the seeds. Slice each half into four wedges.

3. In a small bowl, mix the honey, rosemary, and olive oil.

4. Lay the squash on a greased baking sheet and sprinkle each slice with the honey mixture and sea salt. Turn and sprinkle the other side.

5. Bake for about 30 minutes, until the squash is tender and slightly caramelized, turning each slice halfway through. Serve immediately.

Stuffed Bell Peppers

Makes 6 Servings

Red bell peppers have more nutrients than green or yellow peppers, including plenty of vitamin C and carotenoids, and their nutritional value is best when they are not subjected to high heat. If you've already had your dairy allowance for the day, simply omit the cheese.

- ¾ cup feta cheese
- ½ cup low-salt olives, pitted
- ½ cup plain, unsweetened Greek yogurt
- ¼ cup minced onion
- ¼ cup olive oil, plus more for drizzling
- 1 teaspoon dried thyme, finely chopped
- ½ teaspoon dried dill weed
- 6 bell peppers, cored, seeded, and cut in half lengthwise

1. Combine all the ingredients except the bell peppers in a food processor or blender. Pulse for 30 seconds, or until blended.

2. Carefully spoon the mixture into the bell peppers.

3. Refrigerate for up to 4 hours. Drizzle with olive oil before serving.

Swiss Chard with White Beans and Bell Peppers

Makes 4 Servings

Greens and beans are traditionally paired in Italian cuisine. Beans are inexpensive, nutritional powerhouses that fill you up. Use a red bell pepper whenever possible in recipes that call for bell peppers; they are riper and have more nutrients.

- 2 tablespoons olive oil
- 1 medium onion, chopped
- 1 bell pepper, diced
- 2 cloves garlic, minced
- 1 large bunch Swiss chard, tough stems removed and cut into 2-inch pieces
- One 15-ounce can cooked white beans
- Sea salt and freshly ground black pepper

1. Heat the oil in a large skillet over medium-high heat. Add the onion and bell pepper, and cook for 5 minutes until soft.

2. Add the garlic, stir, and add the Swiss chard. Cook for 10 minutes until greens are tender.

3. Add the beans, stir until heated through, and season with sea salt and black pepper. Serve immediately.

Spiced Sweet Potatoes with Peas and Cauliflower

Makes 4–6 Servings

This versatile, easy-to-prepare dish makes a tasty side dish or can star as the main course meal on Meatless Mondays.

- 2 tablespoons coconut oil
- ½ teaspoon salt
- ½ teaspoon ground turmeric
- ¼ teaspoon chili powder
- ¼ teaspoon paprika
- 1 pound sweet potatoes or yams, peeled and cut into ½-inch pieces
- 1 tablespoon minced fresh ginger
- 4 cups cauliflower florets, cut into bite-size pieces
- ½ cup water
- 1 cup frozen peas, thawed
- Sea salt and freshly ground black pepper

1. Heat the coconut oil in large nonstick skillet over medium heat. Add the salt, turmeric, chili powder, and paprika and toast until fragrant, about 30 seconds.

2. Add the sweet potatoes and ginger; sauté until the potatoes are lightly browned, about 5 minutes.

3. Mix in the cauliflower and sauté 5 minutes. Add the water; cover and simmer until the vegetables are tender, about 5 minutes. Add the peas and simmer for 2 minutes. Season with sea salt and black pepper and serve.

Mini Moroccan Pumpkin Cakes

Makes 6 Servings

Pumpkin is served in savory Moroccan tagines. These spicy and savory pan-fried cakes of pumpkin, rice, and walnuts can also be served as a side dish and are a tasty way to get your daily requirement of nuts.

- 2 cups cooked brown rice
- 1 cup pumpkin purée
- ½ cup finely chopped walnuts
- 3 tablespoons olive oil
- ½ medium onion, diced
- ½ red bell pepper, diced
- 1 teaspoon ground cumin
- Sea salt and freshly ground black pepper
- 1 teaspoon hot paprika, or a pinch of cayenne
- Plain, unsweetened Greek yogurt, for topping

1. Combine the rice, pumpkin purée, and walnuts in a large bowl; set aside.

2. In a medium skillet, heat 1 tablespoon of the olive oil over medium heat, add the onion and bell pepper, and cook until soft, about 5 minutes. Add the cumin. Remove from the heat.

3. Add the onion mixture to the rice-pumpkin-walnut mixture. Mix thoroughly and season with sea salt, freshly ground pepper, and paprika.

4. In a large skillet, heat the remaining 2 tablespoons olive oil over medium heat. Form the mixture into 1-inch patties, and add them to the skillet. Cook until both sides are browned and crispy, about 3 minutes per side. Serve with Greek yogurt on the side.

6

FRUITS

Mixed Berry Smoothie

Makes 1 Serving

This recipe is easily doubled or tripled. Play around with different nut milks until you find one with a texture and consistency you like.

- 1 cup frozen mixed berries
- ½ banana, peeled
- ½ cup unsweetened almond milk
- ¼ cup silken tofu or kefir

Combine the berries, banana, almond milk, and tofu in a blender; process until smooth.

Honey and Avocado Smoothie

Makes 2 Servings

Loaded with heart-healthful monounsaturated fats, avocado will definitely fill you up in the morning. While common in savory dishes in the Americas, avocados are used in other parts of the world in sweet drinks and desserts.

- 1½ cups unsweetened almond milk
- 1 large avocado, peeled and pitted
- 2 tablespoons honey

Combine the almond milk, avocado, and honey in a blender; process until smooth and creamy.

Peachy Green Smoothie

Makes 2 Servings

You'll get many servings of fruits and vegetables in one delicious drink with this smoothie. It's perfect for days when cooking for yourself is a challenge. Be sure to use Greek yogurt for extra creaminess.

- 1 cup unsweetened almond milk
- 3 cups kale or spinach
- 1 banana, peeled
- 1 orange, peeled and segmented
- 1 small green apple, cored
- 1 cup frozen peaches
- ¼ cup plain, unsweetened Greek yogurt

Put the ingredients in a blender in the order listed, and process on high until smooth.

Plantains with Greek Yogurt and Honey

Makes 4 Servings

For this dish, you want sweet yellow plantains, which often sport brown blotches, indicating ripe sweetness. You will find plantains in most grocery stores or at a market that serves a Latin American clientele.

- 2 tablespoon olive oil
- 2 yellow plantains, peeled and cut into ¾-inch-thick slices
- ½ cup plain, unsweetened Greek yogurt
- 1 tablespoon honey

1. In a medium nonstick sauté pan, heat the olive oil over medium-high heat until shimmering. Add the plantains and cook until golden, about 5 minutes. Flip and cook for an additional 3 minutes. Remove from the heat.

2. Combine the yogurt and honey in a small bowl. Serve plantains drizzled with yogurt.

Honeydew Melon and Berries

Makes 4 Servings

Cool and refreshing, this summer dessert or snack takes just minutes to prepare. If honeydew melon is unavailable, cantaloupe can be substituted.

- 1 honeydew melon, seeded and cut into 1-inch pieces
- 1 tablespoon fresh lemon juice
- 1 pint blueberries, hulled
- ½ cup chopped fresh mint leaves
- 2 tablespoons honey

1. In a medium bowl, toss the honeydew chunks with the lemon juice. Gently stir in the blueberries and mint leaves. If desired, chill before serving.

2. Spoon the honeydew mixture into sturdy glass tumblers or small serving bowls. Drizzle with honey and serve.

Berries with Balsamic Vinegar and Black Pepper

Makes 4 Servings

Black pepper adds a surprising freshness and the balsamic vinegar brings out the sweetness of the berries. This dish is delicious well served atop fresh greens, or try it with a dollop of unsweetened whipped cream or yogurt for a tasty, low-calorie dessert.

- ¼ cup balsamic vinegar
- 1 tablespoon brown sugar
- ¼ teaspoon freshly ground black pepper

- ½ cup sliced strawberries
- ½ cup blueberries
- ½ cup raspberries

In a small bowl, whisk the vinegar, brown sugar, and pepper until combined. Add the berries, stir to combine, and let rest for 10 minutes.

Grilled Stone Fruit

Makes 2 Servings

Juicy summer fruit provides hydration, in addition to vitamins. These stone fruits are also delicious drizzled with balsamic vinegar, instead of cheese and honey, for a savory side dish.

- 2 peaches, halved and pitted
- 2 plums, halved and pitted
- 3 apricots, halved and pitted
- ½ cup low-fat ricotta cheese
- 2 tablespoons honey

1. Heat the grill to medium. Oil the grates or spray them with cooking spray.

2. Place the fruit cut-side down on the grill and grill for 2 to 3 minutes per side, until lightly charred and soft.

3. Serve warm with the ricotta and drizzle with honey.

Pears with Blue Cheese and Walnuts

Makes 1 Serving

Fruit, cheese, and nuts are a classic combination, for health as well as flavor—walnuts provide a good source of Omega-3 fatty acids, and pears are a good source of fiber. Enjoy this treat as a dessert or healthful snack.

- 1 pear, cored and sliced into 12 slices
- ¼ cup crumbled blue cheese
- 12 walnut halves
- 1 tablespoon honey

Arrange the pear slices on a plate and top with the blue cheese crumbles. Top each slice with 1 walnut half and drizzle with honey.

Apple, Peach, and Acorn Squash "Pie"

Makes 2 Servings

This dish has the flavors of a creamy spiced pumpkin pie without the calories. It makes for a hearty fall breakfast, or it can be served for dessert. It's healthful, easy to make, and keeps in the refrigerator for several days.

- ½ acorn squash, seeded and cut into large chunks
- 2 apples, cored and chopped
- 1 fresh peach, pitted and chopped
- 2 tablespoons honey
- 1 tablespoon freshly grated ginger
- ½ teaspoon ground cinnamon
- ¼ teaspoon ground nutmeg
- Pinch of ground cloves
- ½ cup plain, unsweetened yogurt

1. Place the squash in a medium stockpot with water to a depth of 2 inches. Cover and cook over medium-high heat for 10 minutes, until nearly tender. If needed, cook for a few minutes longer.

2. Add or remove water to bring the depth to about 1 inch. Reduce the heat to medium-low. Add the apples and peaches to the pot; then cover and cook for 5 minutes. Check the squash again; it should be tender and easily pierced with a fork. Continue cooking until it's very tender, being sure to maintain a bit of water in the pot.

3. When the squash is tender, use a fork or tongs to transfer it to a large mixing bowl. Remove the skin with a paring knife and discard. Mash the squash well.

4. Use a slotted spoon to transfer the chopped fruit from the pot and combine them with the squash. Stir in the honey, ginger, cinnamon, nutmeg, and cloves. Stir well to combine, cover the bowl, and chill in the refrigerator for 1 to 2 hours. Stir in the yogurt just before serving.

Baked Apples with Almond Butter and Honey

Makes 4 Servings

Don't bake these tender apples with just dessert in mind. Try them as a side dish alongside a roast turkey. You can even serve them at breakfast with a generous dollop of yogurt.

- 4 Cortland apples or other baking apple, cored but not peeled
- 4 teaspoons almond butter
- 4 teaspoons dried cherries
- 4 teaspoons butter
- ½ cup apple cider
- 4 teaspoons honey

---

1. Preheat the oven to 400°F. Place the apples in a 9-by-13-inch baking pan, and stuff each one with 1 teaspoon almond butter and 1 teaspoon dried cherries. Top each apple with 1 teaspoon of the butter.

2. Add the apple cider to the pan and bake the apples, basting every 5 to 7 minutes until tender, about 25 to 35 minutes. Drizzle each apple with 1 teaspoon honey and serve immediately.

Coconut Date Bars

Makes 8 Bars

Dates are surprisingly high in fiber. Mix in a bit of coconut and toasted pecans, and you have a sweet, satisfying treat with no added sugar.

- 3 tablespoons unsweetened shredded coconut
- 1 pound very soft dates, such as medjool, pitted
- ¼ cup pecans, toasted and coarsely chopped

Sprinkle 2 tablespoons of the coconut over the bottom of an 8-inch square baking dish. Firmly press the dates into the coconut, covering the bottom of the dish. Sprinkle with the remaining coconut and the pecans, gently pressing the topping into the dates. Cut into eight 2-inch squares. The bars can be stored in an airtight container for 2 or 3 days.

Cocoa and Coconut Banana Slices

Makes 1 Serving

Frozen bananas have a creamy consistency that mimics ice cream. Bananas are good for you, too—providing dietary fiber, vitamin C, potassium, and manganese. This dessert makes a healthful snack for adults and kids alike.

- 1 banana, peeled and sliced
- 2 tablespoons unsweetened, shredded coconut
- 1 tablespoon non-alkalized cocoa powder
- 1 teaspoon honey

1. Lay the banana slices on a parchment-lined baking sheet in a single layer.

2. Put the baking sheet in the freezer for about 10 minutes, until the banana slices are firm but not frozen solid.

3. Mix the coconut with the cocoa powder in a small bowl. Roll the banana slices in honey, followed by the coconut mixture. You can either eat immediately or put back in the freezer for a frozen, sweet treat.

Fresh Figs with Chocolate Sauce

Makes 4 Servings

Desserts in the Mediterranean are simple and often fruit based. This easy treat would be a good snack, too. You could also serve it with unsweetened Greek yogurt.

- ¼ cup honey
- 2 tablespoons non-alkalized cocoa powder

- 8 fresh figs

---

1. Combine the honey and cocoa powder in a small bowl, and mix well to form a syrup.

2. Cut the figs in half and place cut-side up on a plate.

3. Drizzle with the syrup and serve.

7

GRAINS, LEGUMES, SEEDS, AND NUTS

Granola, Your Way

Makes 6 Servings

In the 1960s, scientists discovered that the fiber in oats—beta glucan—lowers cholesterol by as much as 23 percent. This granola is a great breakfast for those following a heart-healthful diet. Experiment with other ingredients you like: shredded coconut, flaxseeds or chia seeds, or chopped dried apricots or mangos.

- 4 cups rolled oats
- ⅓ cup honey
- ¼ cup canola oil
- 2 teaspoons pure vanilla extract
- 1 teaspoon ground cinnamon
- 1 cup mixed dried fruit
- 1 cup chopped mixed nuts or seeds, such as walnuts, cashews, pecans, or sunflower seeds

1. Preheat the oven to 300°F.

2. In a large bowl, combine the oats, honey, oil, vanilla, and cinnamon. Spread evenly on a large rimmed baking sheet.

3. Bake for 15 minutes. Stir the oats well, and then bake for another 15 minutes, or until evenly toasted. Let cool to room temperature.

4. Transfer the granola to a large bowl, add the fruit and nuts, and stir thoroughly to combine. Serve immediately or store in an airtight container for up to 2 weeks.

Flaxseed and Cranberry Muffins

Makes 18 Muffins

The tart cranberries in these muffins explode with flavor and are packed with antioxidants. Flaxseeds, best digested when ground, provide essential Omega-3 fatty acids.

- 1½ cups fresh or frozen cranberries
- 1 cup whole-wheat flour
- 1 cup buckwheat flour
- 1½ teaspoons baking powder
- ½ teaspoon baking soda
- ¼ teaspoon salt
- ½ cup chopped walnuts or pecans
- ¼ cup (2 ounces) egg whites
- ¼ cup brown rice syrup
- ¼ cup maple syrup
- ⅓ cup canola oil
- 2 teaspoons pure vanilla extract
- ¾ cup fresh orange juice
- 2 tablespoons freshly grated orange zest
- ⅓ cup ground flaxseeds

1. Preheat the oven to 350°F. Coat 18 muffin cups with cooking spray or line with paper liners.

2. Pulse the cranberries in a food processor until coarsely chopped.

3. In a large bowl, mix the whole-wheat flour, buckwheat flour, baking powder, baking soda, salt, and ¼ cup of the nuts; whisk to blend.

4. Whisk the egg whites, brown rice syrup, maple syrup, canola oil, vanilla, orange juice, and orange zest in a medium bowl. Add to the flour mixture, and mix with a rubber spatula just until the dry ingredients are moistened. Fold in the cranberries. Scrape the batter into the prepared pan, spreading evenly. Sprinkle the muffins with the remaining ¼ cup nuts.

5. Bake until the tops are golden and a wooden skewer inserted in the center of a muffin comes out clean, 15 to 18 minutes. Immediately after the muffins come out of the oven, sprinkle with the ground flaxseeds. Cool in the pan on a wire rack for 10 minutes. Loosen the edges and turn the muffins onto the rack to cool completely.

Banana-Blueberry Muffins

Makes 12 Muffins

These muffins have 4 grams of protein and 3 grams of fiber. To boost the number, use regular whole-wheat flour. The muffins will have a denser texture. Serve with trans-fat-free margarine.

- ¾ cup cultured buttermilk or kefir
- ¼ cup brown rice syrup
- ¼ cup honey
- ¼ cup canola oil
- ½ cup (4 ounces) egg whites
- 1 cup (about 3 medium) ripe bananas, mashed
- 1¼ cups whole-wheat pastry flour
- 1 cup all-purpose flour
- 1½ teaspoons baking powder
- ¾ teaspoon ground cinnamon
- ½ teaspoon baking soda
- ½ teaspoon salt
- ¼ teaspoon ground nutmeg
- 1¼ cups blueberries, fresh or frozen

1. Preheat the oven to 400°F. Coat 12 muffin cups with cooking spray or line with paper liners.

2. Whisk the buttermilk, brown rice syrup, honey, oil, and egg whites in a large bowl. Stir in the mashed bananas.

3. Whisk the whole-wheat pastry flour, all-purpose flour, baking powder, cinnamon, baking soda, salt, and nutmeg in a medium bowl.

4. Fold the dry ingredients into the wet ingredients and stir until just combined. Fold in the blueberries. Divide the batter among the prepared muffin cups (they will be full).

5. Bake until the tops are golden brown and a wooden skewer inserted in the center of a muffin comes out clean, 20 to 25 minutes. Cool in the pan for 10 minutes; then remove and let cool on a wire rack for at least 5 minutes more before serving.

Breakfast Rice

Makes 6 Servings

Think of this as your new rice cereal. The combination of fiber, protein, and fat in this dish will keep you satisfied and energized all morning long. Make extra rice the night before to make preparation even faster in the morning.

- ¼ cup olive or canola oil
- 4 scallions, thinly sliced
- 3½ cups cooked brown or wild rice
- 1 tablespoon untoasted sesame oil
- 1 tablespoon rice wine vinegar
- 1 tablespoon wheat-free tamari
- One 5-ounce package chopped kale or baby spinach
- 2 egg whites (½ cup or 4 ounces)
- Salt

1. In a large, nonstick skillet heat the oil over medium-high heat until shimmering. Add the scallions and cook over medium heat until tender, about 2 to 3 minutes. Stir in the cooked brown rice, sesame oil, vinegar, and tamari, and cook until rice is heated through, about 3 minutes. Add the kale and cook until wilted, 2 to 3 minutes longer.

2. Push the cooked rice mixture to the sides of the skillet, and add the egg whites to the middle, stirring until cooked, about 2 minutes. Mix the eggs with the rice. Season with salt and serve.

Mango Sticky Rice

Makes 4–6 Servings

If you cannot find glutinous rice, any short-grain white rice will do for this classic Asian dessert.

- 2 cups glutinous rice
- 1 cup warm water
- One 15-ounce can whole coconut milk

- 2 large mangos, pitted and sliced

1. Soak the rice in the warm water in a microwave-safe bowl for 10 minutes. The rice should begin to look translucent. Place the bowl in the microwave, cover with a plate, and cook on high for 3 minutes. Stir and check to see if the rice has turned translucent. If not, cook for an additional 3 minutes.

2. Meanwhile, in a medium saucepan over low heat, warm the coconut milk. Add the warm coconut milk to the cooked rice and stir to combine. Serve with the mango slices.

Coconut Rice Pudding

Makes 4 Servings

Coconut milk makes this rice pudding extra creamy. Don't save it for dessert. It also makes a nutritious breakfast.

- 1 tablespoon orange-infused olive oil or plain olive oil
- 1 cup cooked long-grain rice
- 1 cinnamon stick
- 1 teaspoon pure vanilla extract
- 1 cup coconut milk unsweetened
- ½ cup flaxseed or hemp milk, plus more as needed
- ½ cup raisins
- ½ cup toasted almonds or pecans
- Pinch of ground nutmeg

1. In a medium sauté pan, heat the olive oil over medium heat until warmed.

2. Add the cooked rice, cinnamon stick, vanilla, and coconut milk and stir to combine. Bring to a simmer and cook, partially covered over low heat, until the coconut milk is absorbed, about 20 minutes.

3. Remove from the heat. Add the flaxseed milk, raisins, almonds, and nutmeg. Let rest, covered, for 10 minutes before serving. Add more flaxseed milk if needed to achieve the desired consistency.

Dolmas Wraps

Makes 3 Wraps

Dolmas—stuffed vegetable dishes—are found in the deli section of most supermarkets.

- ½ cup salad greens, chopped
- ¼ cup chopped cucumber
- ¼ cup chopped tomato
- ¼ cup plain, unsweetened yogurt
- 1 tablespoon crumbled feta cheese
- ⅛ teaspoon garlic powder
- 3 whole-wheat wraps, such as tortillas or lavash
- 3 prepared dolmas

1. Combine the salad greens, cucumber, tomato, yogurt, feta, and garlic powder in a small bowl.

2. To serve, spread the mixture on the whole-wheat wraps, top each with a dolma, and roll.

Tabbouleh

Makes 4 Servings

There are myriad versions of this traditional Middle Eastern salad that is usually made with bulgur. Bulgur is derived from durum wheat, and though it is whole grain, it can cause digestive issues, brain fogginess, and bloating. This gluten-free tabbouleh makes use of quinoa, a fine substitute for the bulgur.

- ½ cup whole-grain quinoa
- 3 tablespoons olive oil
- 1 cup boiling water
- 2 cups finely chopped fresh, flat-leaf parsley
- ½ cup finely chopped fresh mint
- 2 medium tomatoes, cut into ¼-inch-thick slices
- ½ seedless cucumber, peeled, cored, and cut into ¼-inch-thick slices
- 3 tablespoons fresh lemon juice
- ¾ teaspoon salt
- ¼ teaspoon freshly ground black pepper

1. Stir together the quinoa and 1 tablespoon of the olive oil in a heatproof bowl. Pour the boiling water over the quinoa; cover the bowl tightly with plastic wrap and let stand 20 minutes. Drain in a sieve, pressing on the quinoa to remove any excess liquid.

2. Spread the quinoa on a half-sheet pan and allow to cool and dry for about 20 minutes before proceeding.

3. Transfer the quinoa to a bowl and toss with the remaining 2 tablespoons olive oil and the remaining ingredients, remaining ingredients, until combined well. Serve.

Hot Quinoa Breakfast Cereal with Fruit and Flaxseeds

Makes 4 Servings

Look for quinoa in the bulk section of natural foods stores or in the cereal aisle or gluten-free section of your favorite market. Flaked quinoa, which contains the endosperm and the bran, is considered whole grain and provides the same nutritional benefits as whole-grain quinoa and cooks in just under 1 minute with boiling water. If using flaked quinoa, boil water, add to quinoa, stir, and let rest 1 minute before proceeding with step 2.

- 2 cups water
- 1 cup quinoa
- ¼ cup coarsely chopped dried apricots
- Pinch of salt
- 1 tablespoon dried currants
- ½ teaspoon ground cinnamon
- ⅛ teaspoon ground nutmeg
- 1 tablespoon flaxseed oil

1. Bring the water to a rolling boil. Add the quinoa, apricots, and salt. Return to a boil; then simmer gently for about 20 minutes or until the water is completely absorbed. Remove from the heat.

2. Stir in the currants; allow to rest for 5 minutes.

3. Stir in the cinnamon, nutmeg, and oil. Adjust seasonings as needed and serve.

Quinoa Salad with Vegetables and Toasted Pecans

Makes 4 Servings

Fresh vegetables and herbs weave color throughout this dish, and a simple vinaigrette holds it together. Quinoa is perfect for experimenting with: use this recipe as a starting point and then modify it to try different vegetables, nuts, and dried fruits in whatever combinations please you. This dish will keep in the refrigerator for a day or two, developing even more flavor. Bring it to room temperature, drizzle on a little more olive oil to rehydrate, and serve.

For the quinoa:

- 2 tablespoons olive oil
- 2 cups quinoa
- 4½ cups low-sodium chicken broth
- ½ cup whole pecans
- ½ cup finely shredded carrot
- ½ cup finely diced zucchini

- 1 cup halved cherry tomatoes
- ¼ cup dried currants

For the vinaigrette:

- ¼ cup fresh lemon juice
- 2 tablespoons minced shallot
- Freshly ground black pepper
- ¾ cup olive or walnut oil

To make the quinoa:

1. Heat the olive oil in a large frying pan over medium-high heat. Add the quinoa and toast, stirring frequently, for 2 to 3 minutes. Be sure to watch closely, as it can burn quickly.

2. In a large pot, bring the chicken broth to a boil and add the toasted quinoa. Simmer for 15 to 17 minutes, adding water to the pot as needed. Drain and transfer to a large bowl.

3. Meanwhile, in a small frying pan set over medium-high heat, toast the pecans. Stir frequently to keep them from scorching and remove immediately from heat once crisp, as they can burn quickly.

continued ▶

Quinoa Salad with Vegetables and Toasted Pecans *continued* ▶

4. Add the pecans, carrot, zucchini, tomatoes, and currants to the quinoa and mix thoroughly.

To make the vinaigrette:

1. Whisk together the lemon juice and shallot in a small bowl. Season with pepper. Drizzle the oil into the mixture in a thin stream, whisking constantly.

2. Pour the vinaigrette over the quinoa and vegetables, and toss thoroughly. Serve immediately.

Farro Bean Soup

Makes 8 Servings

This soup is an easy and inexpensive introduction to farro, an ancient form of wheat. It is easier to digest than modern wheat because of its lower levels of gluten and is digested slowly to help keep blood sugar levels stable. Find traditional Italian farro or German emmer wheat at a health food store or a specialty foods store.

- 2 tablespoons olive oil
- 1 medium onion, diced
- 1 celery stalk, diced
- 2 garlic cloves, minced
- 8 cups chicken broth or water
- 1 cup white beans, soaked overnight, rinsed, and drained
- One 15-ounce can diced tomatoes, with juice
- 1 cup farro
- ½ teaspoon dried thyme
- Sea salt and freshly ground black pepper

1. Heat the olive oil in a large stockpot over medium-high heat.

2. Sauté the onion, celery, and garlic until tender, about 8 minutes.

3. Add the chicken broth, beans, tomatoes, farro, and thyme and bring to a simmer.

4. Cover and cook for 2 hours, or until the beans and farro are tender.

5. Season with sea salt and black pepper.

Cold Soba Noodles with Peanut Sauce

Makes 4 Servings

Look for soba noodles that have buckwheat as the first ingredient or are 100 percent buckwheat. For the peanut sauce, buy creamy natural peanut butter with no sugar or salt added and the oil separated out.

For the noodles:

- One 8-ounce package organic soba noodles
- 1 red bell pepper, sliced into thin strips
- 2 cups small broccoli florets
- 1 small bunch scallions, thinly sliced
- 1 cup fresh cilantro leaves

For the peanut sauce:

- ½ cup unsweetened coconut milk
- 1 cup creamy natural peanut butter
- 1 tablespoon fresh lime juice
- Chopped unsalted peanuts, for garnish
- 4 sprigs fresh cilantro, for garnish

To make the noodles:

1. Cook the noodles in a large pot of boiling water, according to package instructions. Drain in a colander and run cold water over them to stop the cooking. Set aside and cover with a damp towel.

2. Spray a large frying pan with cooking spray and place over medium-high heat. When the pan is hot, add the bell pepper and sauté until soft, about 5 minutes. Transfer to a bowl and set aside. Spray the pan again and sauté the broccoli until the florets are bright green but still firm, about 3 to 5 minutes. Add to the bowl with the bell pepper.

3. Put the cooled noodles in a large bowl, add the cooked vegetables, and toss well. Stir in the scallions and cilantro.

To make the peanut sauce:

1. Add the coconut milk, peanut butter, and lime juice to a blender or food processor. Process until smooth.

2. Pour the sauce over the noodles and toss well to combine. Divide the noodles among four bowls, sprinkle with lime juice, garnish with the peanuts and cilantro sprigs, and serve.

Cornmeal Halva

Makes 4 Servings

Halva is traditionally made with semolina; this version replaces the wheat with cornmeal. For easier slicing, place the prepared halva in the freezer for at least 15 minutes.

- 1¾ cup hemp milk
- 3 tablespoons rosewater
- 1 teaspoon almond extract
- ½ teaspoon ground cardamom or nutmeg
- ¼ cup agave nectar
- 1 cup coarse cornmeal
- 1 tablespoon slivered almonds

1. Heat the hemp milk, rosewater, almond extract, cardamom, and agave nectar in a saucepan over medium heat until warm, about 5 minutes. Add the cornmeal and cook, stirring continuously, until the mixture has thickened.

2. Spoon into a 9-by-13-inch baking pan. Cool to room temperature. Mix in the almonds and serve.

Classic Hummus

Makes 6–8 Servings

Hummus, a creamy and delicious dip, can be served as an appetizer, as a party food, or just as a snack. Try using hummus in place of mayonnaise on sandwiches.

- Two 15-ounce cans cooked chickpeas, drained and slightly warmed
- ¼ cup olive oil
- Juice of 2 lemons
- 2 or 3 garlic cloves, coarsely chopped
- ¾ cup wheat-free tahini
- ¼ teaspoon sea salt
- ¼ teaspoon freshly ground black pepper
- ½ cup pine nuts, toasted (optional)
- ¼ cup chopped fresh, flat-leaf parsley, for garnish

1. Add the chickpeas, olive oil, lemon juice, and garlic to a food processor and purée until smooth.

2. Add the tahini, salt, and pepper, and continue to blend until creamy. If too thick, a bit of water or olive oil can be used to thin the mixture.

3. Place the hummus in a bowl and top with pine nuts, if desired. Garnish with the chopped parsley.

Cannellini Beans with Mint and Parsley

Makes 6–8 Servings

Any white or heirloom white bean works in this recipe. Feel free to change the herbs with the seasons. Serve with the lamb kebob recipe on page 111.

- ¼ cup olive oil
- ¼ cup chopped fresh mint
- ¼ cup chopped fresh parsley
- ¼ teaspoon sea salt

- 1 anchovy, minced (optional)
- 1 garlic clove, minced (optional)
- Two 15-ounce cans cannellini beans or other prepared white bean, drained and rinsed

In a medium bowl, combine the olive oil, mint, parsley, and salt. Add the anchovy and garlic, if desired. Fold the beans into the herb mixture and serve.

Black Bean and Pineapple Stew

Makes 6 Servings

Make it island-style by adding julienned strips of low-salt ham as a garnish.

- 1 tablespoon canola oil
- 1 large onion, chopped
- 2 carrots, sliced into rounds
- 1 jalapeño chile, stemmed, seeded, and finely diced
- 4 garlic cloves, minced or pressed
- One 15-ounce can diced, fire-roasted tomatoes
- Two 16-ounce cans black beans, rinsed and drained
- 2 cups low-sodium vegetable broth
- 1 tablespoon ancho chili powder
- 1 teaspoon ground cumin
- 2 teaspoons dried Mexican oregano
- 1 pound yellow squash or zucchini
- 1 cup crushed pineapple and juice

1. Heat a Dutch oven or soup pot over medium-high heat and add the canola oil. Add the onion and carrots and cook, stirring, until golden and beginning to brown, about 8 minutes. Add the jalapeño and cook until softened, about 2 minutes. Add the garlic, stir briefly, and then add the tomatoes, black beans, vegetable broth, chili powder, cumin, and oregano. Bring to a boil; then reduce heat and simmer for 15 minutes.

2. While the beans are cooking, trim the squash and cut into 1-inch cubes.

3. Add the squash and pineapple and juice to the stew, increase the heat to medium, and cover. Simmer until squash is just tender, about 6 minutes. Check seasonings, adding more to taste if needed, and serve.

Chili with White Beans

Makes 6–8 Servings

Small in size and delicate in flavor, Great Northern beans have a smooth texture that makes them ideal additions to stews and casseroles. Navy or cannellini beans can be substituted for them in a pinch.

- 1 tablespoon canola oil
- 1½ cups chopped onion
- Two 4-ounce cans chopped green chiles
- 1 teaspoon dried oregano
- 1 teaspoon ground cumin
- ⅛ to ¼ teaspoon cayenne pepper

- Three 15-ounce cans Great Northern beans, rinsed and drained
- 4 cups chicken broth
- 4 cups diced cooked skinless turkey or chicken
- 2 tablespoons cider vinegar

1. Heat the canola oil in a large pot or Dutch oven over medium-high heat. Add the onion; cook, stirring occasionally, until softened, about 5 minutes.

2. Stir in the chiles, oregano, cumin, and cayenne pepper. Cook, stirring occasionally, for 5 minutes. Stir in the beans and chicken broth; bring to a simmer. Cook, stirring occasionally, for 20 minutes.

3. Add the turkey and cider vinegar; cook for 5 minutes more. Serve.

Yellow Dal with Split Peas

Makes 4 Servings

Dal, sometimes spelled dahl, *is a staple of Indian vegetarian cuisine. The color gets an aromatic burst from the turmeric. The cayenne here can really pack some heat, so taste before adding more. To make the soup a bit sweeter, swap 1 cup of the water for 1 cup of fresh orange juice. Serve with a green salad and wild rice.*

- 1 cup dried yellow split peas
- 2 cups water or vegetable broth
- 1 teaspoon ground turmeric
- ¼ teaspoon cayenne pepper
- ½ teaspoon sea salt
- 1 tablespoon margarine
- 1 onion, chopped
- 1½ teaspoons ground cumin
- 2 whole cloves

1. In a large pot, add the split peas and the water and bring to a slow simmer. Add the turmeric, cayenne pepper, and salt and cover. Cook for at least 20 minutes, stirring occasionally.

2. In a large sauté pan, warm the margarine over medium-high heat. Add the onion, cumin, and cloves. Cook for 4 to 6 minutes, until the onion is soft. Add the onion mixture to the split pea pot. Simmer for at least 5 minutes more. Remove the cloves and serve.

Rice and Lentil Salad

Makes 4–6 Servings

With extra rice on hand, this recipe comes together in a snap.

- 2 tablespoons olive oil
- 2 tablespoons sherry vinegar or red wine vinegar
- 1 tablespoon finely chopped shallot
- 1 tablespoon Dijon mustard
- ½ teaspoon paprika, preferably smoked
- ¼ teaspoon sea salt
- ¼ teaspoon freshly ground black pepper
- 2 cups cooked brown rice
- One 15-ounce can lentils, rinsed, or 1⅓ cups cooked
- 1 carrot, diced
- 2 tablespoons chopped fresh, flat-leaf parsley

Whisk the olive oil, sherry vinegar, shallot, mustard, paprika, salt, and pepper in a large bowl. Add the rice, lentils, carrot, and parsley. Stir to combine and serve.

Black-Eyed-Pea Burgers

Makes 4 Servings

Mushrooms are moist, tender, and loaded with umami, the key "fifth" taste that makes so many flavors more appealing. Instead of mashing the black-eyed peas by hand, you can add the pea mixture to the food processor and pulse a few times until coarsely ground before proceeding.

- 5 tablespoons grape-seed or olive oil
- 6 medium cremini mushrooms, cleaned, stemmed, and sliced ¼ inch thick
- ¼ teaspoon dried thyme
- 2 medium garlic cloves, minced
- ½ red onion, chopped
- One 15-ounce can black-eyed peas, drained and rinsed
- 2 tablespoons finely chopped fresh basil or parsley
- ½ teaspoon wheat-free tamari
- 4 lettuce leaves or spelt bread, for serving
- 1 avocado, sliced

1. Heat 3 tablespoons of the olive oil in a large frying pan over medium heat until shimmering. Add the mushrooms and thyme and cook, stirring occasionally, until browned, about 2 to 3 minutes. Add the garlic and red onion, and cook until fragrant and softened, about 2 minutes. Remove from the heat.

2. Place the black-eyed peas in a large bowl and mash with the back of a spoon or a potato masher, leaving a few of the peas intact. Add the mushroom mixture, basil, and tamari and mix until combined. Form the mixture into four patties.

3. Heat the remaining 2 tablespoons oil in a sauté pan over medium-high heat until shimmering. Add the patties and fry until browned, 5 to 6 minutes per side. Serve on lettuce leaves with the avocado slices.

Salted Almonds

Makes 1 Cup

These almonds are easy to prepare and make a great party snack. High in healthful fats, almonds provide manganese, vitamin E, magnesium, and more. They are often served alongside tapas in Spain.

- 1 cup raw almonds
- 1 egg white (2 ounces), beaten
- ½ teaspoon coarse sea salt

1. Preheat the oven to 350°F.

2. Spread the almonds in an even layer on a baking sheet. Bake for 20 minutes, until lightly browned and fragrant. Remove from the oven.

3. Place the almonds in a small, heatproof bowl. Coat the almonds with the egg white and sprinkle with the salt.

4. Return the almonds to the baking sheet and bake for about 5 minutes, until they are dry.

5. Cool completely before serving.

Roasted Mixed Nuts with Tamari

Makes About 4½ Cups

To lighten up this snack, mix with seasoned organic popcorn.

- Coconut oil or canola oil for greasing trays
- 1 cup peanuts
- 1 cup cashews
- 1 cup almonds
- ½ cup pumpkin seeds
- ½ cup sunflower seeds
- ½ cup hazelnuts
- ½ cup macadamia nuts
- ½ cup wheat-free tamari

1. Preheat the oven to 275°F.

2. Lightly grease two baking trays with coconut or canola oil.

3. Add the nuts and seeds to a large bowl. Add the tamari and toss to coat.

4. Allow to rest for 10 minutes; then spread evenly on the prepared baking sheets.

5. Bake for 20 to 25 minutes. Cool completely before serving.

Almond-Honey Power Bars

Makes 8 Bars

The whole-grain cereal and nuts in these bars will help you feel full all morning.

- Olive oil or olive-oil cooking spray
- 1 cup old-fashioned rolled oats
- ¼ cup slivered almonds
- ¼ cup sunflower seeds
- 1 tablespoon flaxseeds, preferably golden
- 1 tablespoon sesame seeds
- 1 cup unsweetened whole-grain puffed cereal

- ⅓ cup dried cranberries
- ⅓ cup chopped dried apricots
- ⅓ cup chopped golden figs
- ¼ cup creamy almond butter
- ¼ cup turbinado sugar or brown sugar
- ¼ cup honey
- ½ teaspoon pure vanilla extract
- ⅛ teaspoon salt

---

1. Preheat the oven to 350°F. Coat an 8-inch square pan with olive oil.

2. Spread the oats, almonds, sunflower seeds, flaxseeds, and sesame seeds on a large, rimmed baking sheet. Bake until the oats are lightly toasted and the nuts are fragrant, shaking the pan halfway through, about 10 minutes. Transfer to a large bowl. Add the puffed cereal, cranberries, apricots, and figs; toss to combine.

3. Combine the almond butter, sugar, honey, vanilla, and salt in a small saucepan. Heat over medium-low heat, stirring frequently, until the mixture bubbles lightly, 2 to 5 minutes.

4. Immediately pour the almond butter mixture over the dry ingredients and mix with a spoon or spatula until no dry patches remain. Transfer to the prepared pan. Lightly coat your hands with cooking spray and press the mixture down firmly to make an even layer (wait until the mixture cools slightly if necessary). Refrigerate until firm, about 30 minutes; cut into 8 bars.

Muhammara

Makes About 2½ Cups

Muhammara is a walnut appetizer or dip common in Turkey and other parts of the Middle East. Many Muhammara recipes call for garlic or bread crumbs, but you will not miss them in this version.

- 3 red bell peppers
- ¾ cup walnuts, crushed
- ½ cup olive oil, plus more if needed
- 1 medium yellow onion, chopped
- 1½ tablespoons chili powder, or 1 fresh Fresno chile, chopped
- ¼ teaspoon ground cumin

1. Preheat the oven to 350°F. Place the whole bell peppers on a greased baking sheet. Roast for about 45 minutes, turning approximately every 15 minutes, until the skin is blackened on all sides.

2. Remove the peppers from the oven, cover with a plate, and let cool. Peel off the skin. Cut open and remove the seeds. Chop the flesh and place in a food processor.

3. Meanwhile, on a separate baking sheet, toast the walnuts for 10 to 12 minutes. Let cool. Add the walnuts to the food processor.

4. In a medium sauté pan, heat the olive oil over medium heat until shimmering. Add the onion and sauté until lightly browned, about 8 minutes. Let cool. Add the sautéed onion to the food processor and blend to a dip consistency.

5. Add the chili powder and cumin and blend, adding more olive oil if needed for the desired consistency.

6. Place the dip in a serving bowl and serve with veggies, or use as a dipping sauce for kebabs.

Hazelnut-Banana Open-Faced Sandwiches

Makes 1 Serving

For a quick lunch or snack, this riff on a peanut butter Sandwich can't be beat.

- 1 tablespoon sugar-free hazelnut-chocolate or roasted hazelnut spread
- 1 slice spelt or millet bread
- ¼ sliced banana

Smooth the hazelnut spread over the bread. Top with banana slices and serve.

Cornmeal Baklava

Makes 6 Servings

No need to work with the difficult phyllo dough. Here is a smooth corn-topping substitute for the phyllo. If you do not have soufflé cups, bake in a 9-inch baking pan.

For the filling:
- ½ cup olive oil
- ½ cup honey
- 1 tablespoon fresh lemon juice
- ½ teaspoon ground cinnamon
- 1 cup chopped walnuts
- 1 cup chopped almonds
- ½ cup golden raisins

For the topping:
- ⅓ cup stone-ground cornmeal (such as polenta)
- ⅓ cup masa harina
- 1 teaspoon baking powder
- ¼ teaspoon sea salt
- 1 teaspoon honey
- ⅓ cup unsweetened almond milk
- 2 teaspoons olive oil or almond oil
- 1 egg white (2 ounces)
- 1 mashed banana

To make the filling:

1. In a small saucepan, gently heat olive oil over low heat. Stir in honey, lemon juice, and cinnamon. Increase heat to medium and cook, stirring occasionally, until mixture is thickened, about 15 minutes. Remove from the heat.

2. Combine thickened honey mixture, walnuts, almonds, and raisins in a small bowl; mix well. Cool to room temperature, about 1 hour.

3. Preheat the oven to 350°F.

continued ▶

Cornmeal Baklava *continued* ▶

To make the topping:

1. In a large mixing bowl, mix the cornmeal, masa harina, baking powder, and salt.

2. In a small bowl, mix the honey, almond milk, olive oil, egg white, and banana until combined.

3. To assemble, in each of six 6-ounce soufflé cups, add 3 tablespoons filling and top with 1 tablespoon topping.

4. Bake for 10 to 15 minutes or until topping begins to brown. Remove from the oven, let cool slightly, and serve.

8

FISH AND SEAFOOD

Salmon Poke

Makes 2 Servings

Poke (pronounced poh-keh)*, a Hawaiian dish similar to sushi, is a terrific, often overlooked source of Omega-3 fatty acids. The crispy skin adds great texture to the dish.*

- ½ pound fillet sushi-grade wild Alaskan sockeye salmon, skin on
- 2 teaspoons wheat-free tamari
- 2 teaspoons sesame oil
- 1 tablespoon toasted sesame seeds
- ¼ teaspoon sea salt
- 3 scallions, finely chopped

---

1. Preheat the oven to 350°F.

2. Fillet the salmon to remove the skin (or ask your fish monger to do it for you) and set the skin aside.

continued ▶

Salmon Poke *continued* ▶

3. Cut the salmon into ½-inch dice and put the pieces into a large mixing bowl.

4. Line a baking sheet with foil or parchment paper and add the skin, scales-side up. Bake until crispy, about 20 minutes. Cool and then cut into thin strips.

5. Drizzle the salmon with the tamari and sesame oil and toss to combine. Add the toasted sesame seeds, salt, and scallions.

6. Sprinkle with the crispy salmon skin and serve.

Salmon Tartare

Makes 4 Servings

If you enjoy the flavors of beef tartare, try this oceanic version. Serve with spelt or flaxseed crackers.

- 1 pound fillet sushi-grade wild Alaskan sockeye salmon, skinless, or smoked wild Alaskan salmon, cut into 1-inch cubes
- Juice of 1 lemon
- 2 teaspoons wheat-free tamari
- 2 teaspoons chopped fresh parsley
- 2 teaspoons chopped capers
- 2 teaspoons chopped cornichons
- 2 teaspoons chopped red onion
- 3 cups baby arugula or mixed lettuce

Place the salmon in a large mixing bowl. Add the lemon juice, tamari, parsley, capers, cornichons, and red onion. Toss gently to combine and serve over lettuce.

Grilled Salmon with Spicy Yogurt

Makes 2–4 Servings

Harissa, a spicy chili sauce from Tunisia, gives this grilled salmon an extra kick.

- 2 cups vegetable stock
- 1 cup quinoa
- 2 tablespoons raisins or dried currants
- ¼ cup fresh basil or mint, finely chopped
- 1 teaspoon ground cinnamon
- ¼ teaspoon ground ginger
- 1 tablespoon honey
- 1 tablespoon olive oil
- Two 6-ounce wild Alaskan salmon fillets
- 1 tablespoon harissa
- One 6-ounce container plain, unsweetened Greek yogurt

1. Preheat the grill.

2. In a medium saucepan, add the vegetable stock and bring to a low boil. Add the quinoa and raisins and simmer, covered, for 20 minutes, or until most of the liquid is evaporated. Remove from the heat. Add the basil and cinnamon and stir to combine.

3. In a small bowl, stir the ginger, honey, and olive oil until well combined. Spread evenly over the salmon fillets. Cook the salmon with the grill lid down and without turning until the fish is cooked through, about 8 minutes.

3. Combine the harissa and yogurt. Serve the fish with the quinoa and the spicy yogurt.

Mustard-Crusted Salmon

Makes 4 Servings

Stone-ground mustard makes a nice foil for fatty salmon. Use leftovers to make the next day's lunch.

- 1 tablespoon olive oil
- 1¼ pounds wild Alaskan salmon fillets, skin on, cut into 4 portions
- ⅛ teaspoon sea salt
- Freshly ground black pepper
- ¼ cup reduced-fat sour cream or crème fraîche
- 2 tablespoons stone-ground mustard
- 2 teaspoons fresh lemon juice
- Lemon wedges, for serving

1. Preheat the broiler. Line a broiler pan or baking sheet with foil, then coat it with olive oil.

2. Place salmon pieces, skin-side down, on the prepared pan. Season with salt and pepper. Combine the sour cream, mustard, and lemon juice in a small bowl. Spread evenly over the salmon.

3. Broil the salmon 5 inches from the heat source until it is opaque in the center, 10 to 12 minutes. Serve with lemon wedges.

Balsamic-Glazed Black Pepper Salmon

Makes 4 Servings

To do this dish justice, use the best-quality balsamic vinegar you can find.

- ½ cup balsamic vinegar
- 1 tablespoon honey
- Four 6-ounce wild Alaskan salmon fillets
- Sea salt and freshly ground black pepper
- 1 tablespoon olive oil

1. Heat a cast-iron skillet over medium-high heat.

2. Mix the balsamic vinegar and honey in a small bowl; set aside half.

3. Season the salmon fillets with the salt and pepper, and brush with the balsamic-honey mixture.

4. Add the olive oil to the skillet and sear the salmon fillets, cooking for 3 to 4 minutes on each side until lightly browned and medium rare in the center.

5. Let sit for 5 minutes. Serve with the remaining balsamic-honey dressing.

Mediterranean Tuna Salad Sandwiches

Makes 2 Servings

Usually loaded with high-fat mayonnaise, tuna salad does not often come to mind as a healthful staple. This version is made with Greek yogurt and flavorful roasted peppers, adding taste and moisture without a lot of fat. You can also enjoy the tuna salad without the bread.

- One 6-ounce can U.S.-sourced albacore or skipjack white tuna, packed in olive oil and drained
- 1 roasted red pepper, finely chopped
- ½ small red onion, finely chopped
- 10 low-salt olives, pitted and finely chopped
- ¼ cup plain, unsweetened Greek yogurt
- 1 tablespoon chopped fresh, flat-leaf parsley
- Juice of 1 lemon
- Sea salt and freshly ground black pepper
- 4 slices quinoa, millet, or spelt bread

In a small bowl, combine all of the ingredients except the bread, and mix well. Season with salt and pepper. Toast the bread. Divide the tuna salad between two slices of the toasted bread and top each with one of the remaining slices. Serve immediately.

Grilled Herbed Tuna

Makes 4 Servings

Tuna is a meaty fish that stands up well to grilling. Just be sure to brush the grill grates with oil before adding the fish so it doesn't stick.

- 2 tablespoons olive oil
- 2 tablespoons fresh basil, chopped
- Juice and zest of 1 lemon
- 2 teaspoons fresh cilantro, chopped
- 1 garlic clove, minced
- Sea salt and freshly ground black pepper
- Four 6-ounce U.S.-sourced yellowfin tuna steaks
- 2 tablespoons chopped flat-leaf parsley for garnish

1. Preheat the grill to medium-high.

2. Combine all the ingredients except the fish and parsley in a small bowl.

3. Brush each side of the tuna with the herb mixture, and let marinate for at least 30 minutes in the refrigerator.

4. Grill 8 to 12 minutes depending on thickness, turning halfway through the cooking time.

5. Garnish with chopped parsley, adjust the seasonings if necessary, and serve immediately.

Fish Tacos

Makes 4 Servings

Most cultures around the globe regularly eat fish for breakfast. You can, too. Prepared smoked trout, salmon, or just about any fish works in this recipe, even leftover fish from whatever you cooked the night before. Of course, fish tacos make an excellent quick dinner as well.

- 2 avocados, halved, pitted, and peeled
- 1 small jalapeño chile, seeded and thinly sliced
- 2 tablespoons finely chopped red onion
- 2 tablespoons finely chopped fresh cilantro
- 5 tablespoons fresh lime juice
- Sea salt and freshly ground black pepper
- ½ small head (4 cups) Savoy cabbage, shredded
- 2 tablespoons vegan (eggless) mayonnaise
- Canola oil, for brushing grill
- 1 pound wild Alaskan salmon, Oregon shrimp, U.S.-sourced yellowfin tuna, or other fish
- Tortillas, for serving
- Hot sauce and lime wedges, for serving

1. Preheat the grill. In a medium bowl, mash the avocados, jalapeño, red onion, cilantro, and 3 tablespoons of the lime juice. Season the guacamole with salt and pepper.

2. In a large bowl, toss the cabbage with the mayonnaise and the remaining 2 tablespoons lime juice. Season with salt and pepper.

3. Brush the fish with the canola oil and season with salt and pepper. Grill over medium-high heat until lightly charred and cooked through, about 10 minutes. Transfer the fish to a platter. (If using prepared or smoked fish, skip this step.)

4. To assemble each taco, spread a dollop of guacamole on a tortilla. Top with a piece of fish and a large spoonful of the cabbage slaw. Serve with hot sauce and lime wedges.

Trout and Parma Ham

Makes 2 Servings

The ham adds richness to the trout. If you do not have sage on hand, substitute parsley or basil or another soft herb.

- 4 slices Parma ham
- 4 sage leaves
- 2 trout fillets
- 2 tablespoons olive oil
- Handful fresh parsley, minced, for garnish
- Lemon wedges, for serving

1. Preheat the oven to 350°F.

2. Lay 2 slices of Parma ham horizontally on a work surface, slightly overlapping, and then place a sage leaf in the middle. Lay one trout fillet vertically in the middle to form a cross shape. Place a second sage leaf on top of the fish and drizzle the fillet with 1 tablespoon of olive oil.

3. Roll the ham around the fillet, leaving the ends hanging out, and secure with a wooden skewer. Repeat the process with the second fillet.

4. Place the trout parcels snugly in an oven dish and bake for 15 to 20 minutes. Remove the fish from the oven and sprinkle with the parsley and a squeeze of lemon.

5. Serve the trout with the pan sauce.

Anchovy and Red Pepper Antipasto

Makes 4 Servings

Antipasto *literally means "before the meal." Strong savory flavors are more satisfying than bland crackers and cheese, so you may find yourself eating less. Serve with whole-grain bread sticks or bread toasted with olive oil.*

- Canola oil for the grill
- 4 whole red bell peppers
- 6 ounces anchovies in oil, chopped
- 1 small shallot, finely chopped
- 2 tablespoons capers, rinsed and drained
- 1 cup kalamata olives, pitted
- ½ cup olive oil
- Sea salt and freshly ground black pepper

1. Preheat the grill to medium-high and swab the grill with canola oil.

2. Place the bell peppers on the grill and cook, turning frequently, until the skins are charred, about 3 minutes per side. Place the peppers in a paper bag and allow them to rest for 10 minutes. Once the peppers have cooled, peel the skins under cold water, and then pat dry with paper towels.

3. Combine the anchovies, shallot, capers, olives, and olive oil in a large bowl. Cut the peppers into chunks, removing any seeds and stems, and toss with the anchovy mixture. Season with salt and pepper and serve.

Sardines in Tomato Sauce

Makes 4 Servings

Sardines are plentiful, cheap, and sustainable. Best of all, they're full of Omega-3 fatty acids. Ask your fishmonger to debone and butterfly them for you.

- 3 tablespoons olive oil
- 1 small onion, sliced thinly
- 4 Roma tomatoes, chopped
- Zest of 1 orange
- Sea salt and freshly ground black pepper
- ½ cup white wine
- 2 pounds fresh sardines, deboned and butterflied
- 2 tablespoons spelt or quinoa bread croutons

1. Preheat the oven to 425°F. Brush baking dish with 1 tablespoon of the olive oil. 1 tablespoon olive oil.

2. Heat the remaining 2 tablespoons olive oil in a large skillet. Add the onion, tomatoes, and orange zest, season with sea salt and pepper, and simmer for 20 minutes, or until the mixture thickens and softens.

3. Place half the sauce in the bottom of the baking dish. Stir in the white wine. Set the fish on top, and spread the remaining sauce over the fish.

4. Top with the croutons and bake for 20 minutes. Serve immediately.

Herring with Mustard and Dill Salad

Makes 4 Servings

The familiar flavors of a classic salad dressing get an update from a dash of curry. Look for mayonnaise made with grape-seed or olive oil and without eggs.

For the herring:
- ½ cup water
- Juice of 2 limes
- ½ cup white wine
- 1 teaspoon white peppercorns
- 2 bay leaves
- 1 tablespoon white wine vinegar
- 1 teaspoon salt
- Four 4-ounce herring fillets

For the pasta salad:
- ½ pound cooked whole-grain fusilli

- ½ cup vegan (eggless) mayonnaise
- 1 tablespoon chopped fresh dill
- 1 tablespoon coarse ground mustard
- Juice of ½ lemon
- ½ teaspoon curry paste
- Sea salt and freshly ground black pepper

- Fresh dill sprigs, for garnish
- Lemon wedges, for garnish

To make the herring:

Bring the water, lime juice, white wine, peppercorns, bay leaves, white wine vinegar, and salt to a slow boil in a pan. Turn down the heat to a gentle simmer, add the fish, and poach for about 12 minutes, or until cooked through.

To make the pasta salad:

1. Place the cooked pasta into a large bowl. In another bowl, combine the mayonnaise, dill, mustard, lemon juice, and curry paste, and season with salt and pepper. Add to the bowl with the pasta and stir to coat.

2. Drain the fish and place it on top of the pasta salad. Garnish with dill sprigs and lemon wedges.

Mackerel and Lentil Salad

Makes 4 Servings

This main-dish salad packs a double dose of oily fish. If you are just dipping your toes into the world of oil-rich fish, you can tone down the strength of the fish flavors by leaving out either the mackerel or the anchovy, or substitute walnut oil for the anchovy.

- 2 tablespoons canola oil
- 1 celery stalk, diced
- 2 carrots, diced
- 1 small onion, chopped
- 3 garlic cloves, minced
- 1 cup lentils
- Sea salt
- 1½ cups chicken broth or water, plus more if needed
- 3 ounces smoked or grilled mackerel
- 1 small red onion, sliced vertically
- 4 anchovy fillets, chopped
- Juice of 1 lemon
- ¼ cup chopped fresh, flat-leaf parsley
- ¼ cup olive oil

1. In a medium sauté pan, heat the canola oil over medium heat until shimmering. Add the onion, celery, carrots, and garlic and sauté until vegetables are softened and beginning to brown, about 8 minutes.

2. Add the lentils, sprinkle with salt, and add the chicken broth. Stir to combine. Bring to a low boil and simmer, uncovered, until the lentils are al dente, about 20 minutes. Add more broth, if needed, ¼ cup at a time, to prevent scorching. Remove from the heat.

3. Place the lentils in a large, heatproof salad bowl. Remove the skin from the mackerel.

4. Place the fish on top of the lentils. Add the red onion, anchovy fillets, lemon juice, and parsley. Add the olive oil and mix to combine. Serve.

Grilled Bluefish

Makes 4 Servings

The citrus in this dish lends it a sunny Mediterranean flavor. If you can find small, whole bluefish, clean and grill them whole. Otherwise, fillets work fine. Bluefish is a good source of niacin, phosphorus, selenium, and vitamin B_6 and B_{12}.

- 1 cup olive oil, plus more for greasing grill
- ½ cup white wine
- ¼ cup fresh basil leaves, cut into ¼-inch diagonal slices
- Juice and zest of 2 lemons or oranges
- 2 or 3 garlic cloves, minced
- 1 teaspoon ground cumin
- 1 teaspoon dried thyme
- ⅛ teaspoon cayenne pepper
- 4 small, whole bluefish or fillets
- Sea salt and freshly ground black pepper

1. Combine the olive oil, white wine, basil, lemon zest and juice, garlic, cumin, thyme, and cayenne in a ziplock bag or shallow pan such as a pie plate.

2. Divide the marinade in half, reserving the other half. Place the fish in the marinade and refrigerate, covered, for at least 1 hour.

3. Preheat a grill to medium-high. Brush the grates with olive oil and grill the fish for 6 to 8 minutes, turning halfway through the cooking time. Season with salt and pepper.

4. Warm the reserved marinade and serve with the fish.

Shrimp Soup with Leeks and Fennel

Makes 6 Servings

The Provençal flavors of leek, fennel, garlic, and shrimp are featured in this elegant soup. Low in calories yet filling, this soup provides several servings of vegetables. You can substitute scallops for the shrimp, if you prefer.

- 2 tablespoons olive oil
- 3 stalks celery, chopped
- 1 leek, both white and light green parts, sliced
- 1 medium fennel bulb, chopped
- 1 garlic clove, minced
- Sea salt and freshly ground black pepper
- 1 tablespoon fennel seeds
- 4 cups vegetable or chicken broth
- 1 pound medium shrimp, peeled and deveined
- 2 tablespoons light cream
- Juice of 1 lemon

1. Heat the olive oil in a large Dutch oven over medium heat. Add the celery, leek, and fennel, and cook for about 15 minutes, until the vegetables are browned and very soft.

2. Add the garlic and season with salt and pepper. Add the fennel seeds and stir. Add the broth and bring to a boil. Reduce to a simmer and cook for about 20 minutes.

3. Add the shrimp and cook until just pink, about 3 minutes. Add the cream and lemon juice and serve immediately.

Chili Shrimp

Makes 6 Servings

This tasty and spicy side dish is great for potlucks and other festive occasions.

- ½ cup olive oil
- 5 garlic cloves, minced
- 1 teaspoon red pepper flakes
- 24 large shrimp, peeled and deveined
- Juice and zest of 1 lemon
- Sea salt and freshly ground black pepper

1. Heat the olive oil in a large skillet over medium-high heat.

2. Add the garlic and red pepper flakes and cook for 1 minute.

3. Add the shrimp and cook for 3 minutes, stirring frequently.

4. Remove from the pan and sprinkle with lemon juice, salt, and pepper. Serve hot. Alternatively, cool shrimp to room temperature, then place in the refrigerator to chill.

Mussels in Tomato Sugo

Makes 2 Servings

This dish is a riff on the classic pairing of seafood and tomato. After adding the mussels to the sauce, cook just long enough to warm them through.

- 3 tablespoons olive oil
- 1 onion, finely chopped
- 3 garlic cloves, minced
- 2 tablespoons chopped fresh thyme
- ¾ cup red wine
- One 28-ounce can low-salt peeled and diced tomatoes, liquid reserved

- 2 pounds fresh mussels, cleaned and debearded
- Sea salt and freshly ground black pepper
- 2 tablespoons chopped fresh parsley, for garnish
- Crusty spelt or quinoa bread, for serving (optional)

1. Add the olive oil to a deep sauté pan and heat over medium-high heat until shimmering. Add the onion and sauté until it softens and caramelizes, about 8 minutes.

2. Stir in the garlic and thyme and cook for 1 minute.

3. Add the red wine to the onion mixture, return to a simmer, and cook for 5 minutes.

4. Add the tomatoes, cover, and let simmer for 30 minutes.

5. Add the mussels and a pinch each of salt and pepper and stir to combine. If the tomatoes have reduced too far to evenly coat the mussels, add the reserved liquid, ¼ cup at a time, until the consistency is saucy. Cook the mussels, stirring occasionally, until the shells open, about 4 to 5 minutes.

6. Garnish with parsley and serve with crusty spelt bread, if desired.

Cioppino

Makes 8–10 Servings

Invented in San Francisco, this Italian-American favorite is a delectable medley of seafood and fish. It makes a great dish for company.

- ½ cup olive oil
- 2 medium onions, chopped
- 3 garlic cloves, minced
- 1 bunch fresh parsley leaves, minced
- Two 15-ounce cans diced plum tomatoes, undrained
- Two 8-ounce bottles clam juice
- 2 bay leaves
- 8 sprigs fresh thyme
- 6 sprigs fresh oregano
- 1½ cups white wine
- 12 small clams in shell, cleaned
- 12 mussels in shell, cleaned
- 1½ pounds raw large shrimp, peeled and deveined
- 1 pound fish fillets (such as wild Alaskan salmon), cut into bite-size chunks
- Sliced fresh basil for serving
- Freshly ground white pepper

1. In a large soup pot or Dutch oven, heat the olive oil over medium-low heat. Add the onions, garlic, and parsley. Cook slowly, stirring occasionally, until the onions are softened, about 8 minutes.

2. Add the tomatoes, clam juice, bay leaves, thyme, oregano, and white wine; bring just to a boil, and then reduce heat to low; cover and simmer 45 minutes to 1 hour.

3. Gently stir the clams, mussels, shrimp, and fish fillets into the stock. Cover and simmer 5 minutes, until the clams pop open and the shrimp are opaque when cut. Remove from the heat. Remove the bay leaves and herb stems; season with basil and white pepper and serve.

Curried Seafood

Makes 4 Servings

Most curry recipes call for a bit of sugar to tame the vibrant flavor of the curry. You will not miss the sugar in this version. Any curry paste will work for this dish, including yellow or vindaloo. Look for dry-packed scallops, as these have not been treated with artificial preservatives.

- 2 tablespoons canola oil
- 1½ tablespoon red curry paste
- ½ yellow onion, sliced
- 1 red chile, cut into ¼-inch slices, plus red chile slices for serving
- 5 ounces coconut milk
- ¼ cup water
- 1 kaffir lime leaf cut into fine thin strips, or zest of 1 lime
- 8 ounces scallops
- 8 ounces tiger prawns or shrimp
- ¼ teaspoon fish sauce
- Lime wedges, for serving

1. Heat the canola oil in a medium saucepan or Dutch oven over medium-high heat until shimmering.

2. Add the curry paste and sauté until aromatic, about 1 minute. Add the onion and chile.

3. Add the coconut milk, water, and kaffir lime leaf; bring the curry to a low boil.

4. Add the scallops and the prawns into the pan, and cook gently for 1 to 2 minutes or until the prawns and scallops are cooked. Remove from the heat.

5. Add the fish sauce and stir just to combine. Serve with the chile slices and lime wedges.

9

MEAT AND POULTRY

Grilled Skirt Steak with Salsa Verde

Makes 4 Servings

Marinating the steak adds extra flavor to this zesty dish. Use whatever fresh herbs are in season for the salsa verde.

- 1½ pounds skirt steak
- ½ teaspoon sea salt
- ½ teaspoon freshly ground black pepper
- ¼ cup grape-seed oil
- Zest of 1 lemon
- 2 garlic cloves, minced
- ¼ cup olive oil
- 1 cup minced soft herbs such as mint, tarragon, or basil
- 1 cup minced fresh, flat-leaf parsley
- 2 avocados, cut into ¼-inch dice
- 1 cup kefir or plain, unsweetened Greek yogurt

continued ▶

Grilled Skirt Steak with Salsa Verde *continued* ▶

1. Preheat the grill to medium-high.

2. Season the steak with salt and pepper. In a small bowl, combine the grape-seed oil, lemon zest, and garlic. Place the flank steak in a shallow dish and rub the mixture into the meat. Allow to rest for 20 minutes.

3. Meanwhile, in a medium bowl, combine the olive oil with the herbs and parsley. Stir in the avocado. Stir in the kefir or yogurt, ¼ cup at a time, until the salsa reaches a consistency you like.

4. Grill the steak until charred, about 2 minutes per side for medium rare. Allow to rest before slicing. Serve with the salsa.

Zesty Grilled Flank Steak

Makes 6 Servings

Flank steak, a lean cut of meat, benefits from a long marinating time. Start marinating the meat the night before, and you're ready to go. Thin slices of lean steak can be served over a salad or pile of fresh vegetables. Make sure you eat a larger portion of vegetables than meat at every meal.

- ¼ cup olive oil
- 3 tablespoons red wine vinegar
- 1 teaspoon dried rosemary
- 1 teaspoon dried marjoram
- 1 teaspoon dried oregano
- 1 teaspoon paprika
- 2 garlic cloves, minced
- 1 teaspoon freshly ground black pepper
- 2 pounds flank steak

1. Combine the olive oil, red wine vinegar, and herbs and seasonings in a small bowl. Place the flank steak in a shallow dish and rub the marinade into the meat. Cover and refrigerate for up to 24 hours.

2. Preheat the grill to medium. Grill the steak for 18 to 21 minutes, turning once halfway through. An internal meat thermometer should read 135°F to 140°F when the steak is cooked to medium-rare.

3. Transfer the steak to a cutting board and tent with aluminum foil. Let the steak rest for at least 10 minutes. Slice thinly against the grain and serve.

Greek Beef Kebabs

Makes 6 Servings

Olive oil, lemon, oregano, garlic, and bay leaves are classic Greek seasonings. Lean meat like sirloin beef is a good source of protein you can enjoy a few times a week on this diet. Serve the kebabs with grilled vegetables.

- ¼ cup olive oil
- Juice of 1 lemon
- 1 tablespoon dried oregano
- 2 garlic cloves, minced
- 5 bay leaves
- Sea salt and freshly ground black pepper
- 2 pounds beef sirloin, cut into 2-inch cubes

1. Combine all the ingredients except the beef cubes in a ziplock bag. Add the beef and shake to coat. Marinate for up to 24 hours and drain.

2. Preheat a grill to medium-high. Skewer the meat onto 8-inch skewers and grill on medium heat for 8 to 10 minutes, turning the skewers halfway through the cooking time.

Lamb Kebabs with Garlic and Mint

Makes 4–6 Servings

The heartiness of the anchovy works beautifully with lamb. Serve with the cannellini bean recipe on page 74.

- 2 anchovies
- 2 garlic cloves, minced
- ¼ teaspoon sea salt
- 3 tablespoons plus ¼ cup olive oil
- 2 pounds lamb leg, cut into 2-inch cubes
- ¼ cup chopped fresh mint

1. Mash together the anchovies, garlic, and salt until a coarse paste forms. Add the paste to a medium bowl; then add 3 tablespoons of the olive oil and the cubes of lamb. Mix until the cubes are evenly coated. Let the mixture rest for 30 minutes or up to 2 hours.

2. Preheat the grill to medium-high. When the grill is ready, sear the lamb cubes to medium-rare, about 5 minutes per side.

3. Meanwhile, mix the remaining ¼ cup olive oil and mint in a small bowl.

4. Place the lamb cubes on a serving plate and sprinkle with the mint oil.

Smoky Buffalo Burgers

Makes 6 Servings

A lean red meat, buffalo is raised from start to finish on grass. It is never fed corn or by-products, so its meat has a clean, fresh flavor. Because of its low-fat content, it cooks more quickly than conventional beef burgers. Grill at medium heat.

- 1 pound ground buffalo (American bison)
- 1 teaspoon cracked black pepper
- 1 teaspoon smoked paprika
- 1 teaspoon sea salt
- ½ yellow onion, minced
- ¼ cup smoky barbecue sauce, such as chipotle-honey, plus more for serving
- 12 slices spelt bread
- 6 slices smoked mozzarella cheese

1. Preheat the grill. In a large bowl, combine the ground buffalo, pepper, paprika, salt, minced onion, and barbecue sauce until well mixed. Shape into six patties.

2. Place the patties on the grill and sear about 3 minutes per side. Serve on spelt bread topped with smoked mozzarella cheese and additional barbecue sauce.

Afelia

Makes 6 Servings

Afelia, a classic stew from Cyprus, gets its unique flavor from coriander, cinnamon, and red wine. Serve it with brown rice and a green salad. Any leftovers can be used for sandwiches the next day.

- 2 pounds boneless pork roast, cut into 2-inch pieces
- 1 cup red wine
- 1 tablespoon crushed coriander seeds
- 1 cinnamon stick
- Sea salt and freshly ground black pepper
- ¼ cup olive oil
- 1 cup small white onions, peeled
- 3 bay leaves

1. Place the pork chunks in a shallow bowl. Add the red wine, coriander seeds, and cinnamon stick, cover, and marinate in the refrigerator for several hours or overnight. Strain, reserving the liquid, and pat the pork chunks dry with a paper towel. Season the pork with salt and pepper.

2. Heat the olive oil in a large stew pot or skillet. Add the pork and onions, and cook for 8 to 10 minutes, stirring frequently. Add the bay leaves, salt and pepper, and the reserved liquid. Cover and simmer on low for 2 hours, or until the pork is very tender.

3. Remove the bay leaves, simmer an additional 15 minutes to thicken the sauce, and serve.

Pork Loin in Dried Fig Sauce

Makes 6 Servings

Pork loin, a lean meat, pairs beautifully with fruit or fruity wine. If you can't find dried figs, substitute dried apricots. Both dried figs and dried apricots are high in fiber.

- 3 teaspoons fresh rosemary
- 1 tablespoon fresh thyme
- ½ teaspoon sea salt
- ½ teaspoon freshly ground black pepper
- Two 1½-pound pork loins
- ½ cup olive oil
- 3 carrots, peeled and cut into ½-inch diagonal pieces
- 1 onion, chopped
- 1 garlic clove, minced
- 1 cup dried figs, cut into quarters
- 1 cup white wine
- Juice of 1 lemon

1. Preheat the oven to 350°F.

2. Mix together the rosemary, thyme, and salt and pepper. Rub the mixture into the pork loins.

3. Heat the olive oil in a skillet. Add the pork loin, carrots, onion, and garlic and cook for 4 minutes per side, or until the pork is browned.

4. Transfer all to a shallow 9-by-13-inch roasting pan. Add the figs, white wine, and lemon juice. Cover with aluminum foil and bake for 20 to 30 minutes, or until the meat is tender and the internal temperature is about 145°F.

5. Transfer the meat to a serving dish and cover with aluminum foil. Wait about 15 minutes before slicing.

6. In the meantime, pour the vegetables, figs, and liquids into a blender. Process until smooth and strain through a sieve or strainer. Transfer to a gravy dish, or pour directly over the sliced meat.

Pork Chops with Double Pumpkin

Makes 4 Servings

Pumpkin seed oil, popular in Austrian cooking, turns rancid more quickly than some other oils. Purchase the smallest bottle you can find and store in the refrigerator after opening. If fresh pumpkin is unavailable, you can use other winter squash, such as butternut or delicata, in this recipe.

- 3 pounds pumpkin, halved, seeded, and flesh scooped out and cut into 1-inch wedges
- 4 tablespoons olive oil
- 4 thin-cut pork chops (about 1 pound)
- ¼ cup pumpkin seed oil
- Juice of 1 lemon
- 2 tablespoons minced fresh parsley
- 2 cups arugula or mixed greens
- 2 tablespoon toasted pumpkin seeds

1. Preheat the oven to 425°F. On a rimmed baking sheet, toss the pumpkin wedges with 3 tablespoons of the olive oil. Roast, turning occasionally, until brown in spots and tender, about 30 minutes.

2. Meanwhile, heat a large skillet over medium-high heat and add the remaining 1 tablespoon olive oil. Cook the pork chops until brown, about 4 minutes per side.

3. Whisk together the pumpkin seed oil, lemon juice, and parsley. Divide the pumpkin and pork equally among four plates, top each with a mound of arugula, a sprinkle of pumpkin seeds, and 1 tablespoon of the pumpkin seed oil vinaigrette.

Grilled Chicken Caesar Salad with Cashews

Makes 4 Servings

Egg yolk is replaced here by toasted cashews, which give the dressing a creamy, thick character. If cashews are too sweet for your taste, replace with sunflower seeds.

- Canola oil for the grill
- 1½ pounds boneless skin-on chicken breasts
- ¼ cup toasted cashews or sunflower seeds
- 1 teaspoon anchovy paste
- ¼ cup fresh lemon juice
- 1 garlic clove, minced
- 1 tablespoon spicy brown mustard
- ¼ teaspoon sea salt
- ¼ teaspoon freshly ground black pepper
- 3 tablespoons olive oil
- 12 cups torn romaine lettuce
- 1 tablespoon Parmesan cheese

1. Preheat the grill to medium. Grease the grill with the canola oil. Place the chicken on the grill and cover. Turn after 8 minutes and grill for 15 minutes total, or until the chicken is no longer pink in the center and an internal temperature measures 165°F.

2. Meanwhile, in a blender, blend the cashews, anchovy paste, lemon juice, garlic, mustard, and salt and pepper until combined. Pour the dressing into a small bowl and whisk in the olive oil until emulsified. If the dressing is too thick, add more olive oil, 1 tablespoon at a time, until it reaches the desired consistency.

3. Let the chicken cool for 10 minutes; then cut into strips. Place the lettuce in a large bowl. Add the chicken and mix lightly.

4. Pour the dressing over the salad and toss to coat. Sprinkle with Parmesan and serve immediately.

Coleslaw Chicken Salad with Asian Flavors

Makes 4–6 Servings

The fats in this salad—from oils, almonds, and seeds—create a warmth of flavor that nicely balances the crunch of the cabbage and vegetables. If you desire, you can substitute 1 pound shrimp for the chicken.

For the dressing:
- ½ cup canola oil
- 3 teaspoons sesame oil
- ¼ cup rice vinegar
- 3 tablespoons wheat-free tamari
- 1 tablespoon fresh lime juice
- 2 teaspoons honey
- 2 teaspoons toasted sesame seeds
- 2 teaspoons minced ginger
- 1 garlic clove, minced
- Sea salt and freshly ground black pepper

For the salad:
- 1 small napa or Savoy cabbage (about 1½ pounds), cored and shredded
- 1½ pounds bone-in skin-on chicken breasts, roasted and shredded
- ½ cup loosely packed fresh cilantro leaves
- 3 ounces mung bean sprouts or sunflower seed sprouts
- 10 snow peas, julienned
- 4 scallions, cut into ¼-inch-thick slices
- 1 carrot, julienned
- 1 cucumber, peeled, seeded, and cut into ¼-inch-thick slices
- 1 Thai chile, cut into ¼-inch-thick slices
- ½ cup toasted sliced almonds
- ¼ cup toasted sesame seeds

To make the dressing:
Place all the dressing ingredients in a jar and shake vigorously.

To make the salad:
1. Toss all the salad ingredients together.

2. Serve the salad with the dressing on the side.

Turkey-Spinach Meatloaf

Makes 6 Servings

A painless way to increase your vegetables, this dish combines spinach with ground turkey to create a moist, flavorful meatloaf.

- 3 tablespoons canola oil, plus more if needed
- 2 slices turkey bacon, chopped, plus 4 whole slices
- 1 large onion, chopped
- 1 large carrot, chopped
- 2 garlic cloves, minced
- 1 egg white (2 ounces)
- ¼ cup plain, unsweetened Greek yogurt or sour cream
- ¼ cup unsweetened almond milk
- 2 teaspoons mustard
- ½ teaspoon dried thyme
- ½ teaspoon freshly ground black pepper
- 1 tablespoon wheat-free tamari
- 1 pound ground turkey
- One 10-ounce package frozen spinach, thawed
- ⅓ cup finely chopped fresh flat-leaf parsley

---

1. Preheat the oven to 375°F.

2. In a medium sauté pan, heat the canola oil over medium-high heat. Add the chopped bacon and cook, stirring occasionally, until crisp, about 8 minutes. Remove the bacon with a slotted spoon and reserve. Add a bit more oil to the pan if needed, then add the onion, carrot, and garlic and cook, covered, for about 10 minutes, until the onion and garlic are translucent and just beginning to brown. Remove from the heat.

3. In a medium bowl, whisk together the egg white, yogurt, almond milk, mustard, thyme, black pepper, and tamari.

4. In a large bowl, crumble the ground turkey and add the spinach, onion mixture, chopped bacon, and parsley. Using your hands, shape the mixture into a rectangular loaf. Place the loaf in a baking pan or

rimmed half-sheet pan lined with parchment paper. Drape the 4 turkey bacon slices over the meatloaf.

5. Bake in the center of the oven until the internal temperature reaches 165°F, about 1 hour. Let cool in the pan for about 10 minutes before slicing.

10

DAIRY AND EGGS

Yogurt with Granola and Fruit

Makes 1 Serving

Take advantage of whatever fresh fruit is in season when making this simple yet nourishing breakfast.

- 1 cup plain, unsweetened yogurt
- 2 tablespoons wheat-free granola, such as the granola on page 56
- 2 tablespoons sliced fruit, such as blueberries, apples, pears, or peaches

---

In a small bowl, combine all the ingredients until the granola is moist. Serve immediately.

Versatile Cracker Spread

Makes About 1 Cup

This is a riff on a midcentury classic and can be adapted in myriad ways to suit the day's nutritional needs. Cultured dairy products are more bio-available, meaning the nutrients they contain are more easily absorbed.

- 1 cup crème fraîche or cultured sour cream
- 2 tablespoons flaxseed, olive, or pumpkin seed oil
- 1 tablespoon chopped fresh basil, parsley, mint, or other soft herb (optional)
- 1 tablespoon chopped scallions or chives (optional)
- 1 teaspoon garlic powder (optional)
- 2 ounces smoked salmon, trout, herring, or sardine (optional)
- Endive spears or spelt crackers, for serving

In a small bowl, mix the crème fraîche, oil, and any or all of the optional ingredients until well combined. Serve with endive spears or spelt crackers.

Cheese-and-Ham Corn Cakes

Makes 10–12 Corn Cakes

In Venezuela they make arepas, a corn cake without wheat flour. The taste is of pure corn. With a bit of cheese and ham, these cakes make a handy snack. In Columbia, it is traditional to eat them with a cup of unsweetened hot chocolate (see page 130). Look for arepa flour at Latin grocers or well-stocked specialty stores.

- 1 cup arepa flour (precooked cornmeal, sometimes called *harina de maiz refinada* or *precocida*)
- 1 cup (¼ pound) crumbled queso blanco or aged mozzarella
- ½ cup sliced low-salt ham
- 1 cup plus 2 tablespoons water
- ¼ cup canola or grape-seed oil

1. Toss together the arepa flour, cheese, and ham in a bowl. Stir in the water until incorporated. Let stand until enough water is absorbed for a soft dough to form, 1 to 2 minutes (dough will continue to stiffen). Your dough should be moist but not sticky.

2. Using wet hands, form 3 level tablespoons into a ball and flatten between your palms, gently pressing to form a ¼-inch-thick patty, 2 to 3 inches wide. Gently press the sides to eliminate cracks. Transfer to a wax-paper-lined plate. Keeping hands moist, continue to form more disks with the remaining dough, transferring each disk to the plate.

3. Heat the canola or grape-seed oil in a large nonstick or cast-iron skillet over medium heat until it shimmers. Fry the arepas in two batches, turning once, until deep golden in patches, 8 to 10 minutes per batch. Drain on paper towels.

Strawberries with Lemon Ricotta

Makes 4 Servings

Strawberries are at their sweetest in season. If you are preparing this dish with imported strawberries, allow them to come to room temperature before adding more honey.

- 1 teaspoon pure vanilla extract
- 3 tablespoons honey, or more to taste
- 2 teaspoons white balsamic vinegar
- Pinch of sea salt
- 3 cups strawberries, hulled and quartered
- 2 cups part-skim ricotta cheese
- 2 tablespoons freshly grated lemon zest

1. Add the vanilla, honey, white balsamic vinegar, and salt to a small bowl; whisk until well combined. Add the strawberries and stir to combine. Let stand at room temperature for at least 15 minutes and up to 2 hours, stirring occasionally.

2. Just before serving, combine the ricotta and lemon zest in another bowl.

3. Taste the strawberry mixture; if it's too tart, add a little more honey. To serve, spoon ½ cup of the ricotta into each of four dessert bowls and top each with about ⅓ cup of the strawberry mixture. Serve immediately.

No-Bake Cheesecake

Makes One 9-inch Cake

You'll toss aside any outdated notions about cottage cheese after you taste this delicious no-bake tart. Low-fat ricotta makes a fine alternative to cottage cheese.

- 2 tablespoons water
- 1 envelope unflavored gelatin
- 2 tablespoons orange juice
- ½ cup unsweetened almond or hemp milk, heated almost to boiling
- 2 tablespoons ground flaxseeds
- ¼ cup maple syrup
- 1 teaspoon pure vanilla extract
- 2 cups low-fat cottage cheese
- Freshly grated orange zest (optional)

1. Combine the water, gelatin, and orange juice in the bowl of a food processor or blender. Process on low speed for 1 to 2 minutes to soften the gelatin.

2. Add the hot almond milk, processing until the gelatin is dissolved. Add the flaxseeds, maple syrup, vanilla, and cottage cheese. Process until smooth.

3. Pour into a 9-inch pie plate or round flat dish. Refrigerate for 2 to 3 hours. Top with the orange zest, if desired.

Breakfast Burrito

Makes 2 Servings

Substantial and a snap to prepare, this burrito is an ideal meal to eat on the run. Just be sure to bring along plenty of napkins.

- 2 corn tortillas
- ½ cup (4 ounces) egg whites
- 2 tablespoons shredded reduced-fat Cheddar cheese
- 2 pieces reduced-fat turkey bacon, cooked and chopped
- 1 tablespoon salsa
- ½ sliced avocado

1. Place the tortillas in a nonstick pan and warm gently over low heat.

2. Meanwhile, heat another nonstick pan over medium heat. Add the egg whites and cook, stirring occasionally, until whites are set, about 2 minutes. Divide the egg between the tortillas. Top with cheese, bacon, salsa, and avocado. Serve immediately.

Fresh Veggie Frittata

Makes 1 Serving

You can use whatever vegetables you have on hand for this recipe—grilled or roasted vegetables add great depth of flavor.

- ¾ cup (6 ounces) egg whites
- 1 teaspoon unsweetened almond milk
- 1 tablespoon olive oil
- 1 handful baby spinach leaves
- ½ baby eggplant, peeled and diced
- ¼ small red bell pepper, chopped
- Sea salt and freshly ground black pepper
- 1 ounce crumbled goat cheese

1. Preheat the broiler.

2. Beat the egg whites with the almond milk until just combined.

3. Heat a small nonstick, heatproof skillet over medium-high heat.

4. Add the olive oil, followed by the eggs. Spread the spinach on top of the egg mixture in an even layer, and top with the eggplant and bell pepper.

5. Reduce the heat to medium and season with salt and pepper. Allow the eggs and vegetables to cook without stirring for 3 to 5 minutes, until the bottom of the eggs is firm and the vegetables are tender.

6. Top with the goat cheese and place under the broiler. Cook another 3 to 5 minutes, until the cheese has melted. Slice into wedges and serve immediately.

Egg Drop Soup

Makes 6 Servings

This soup is as nourishing for breakfast as it is for lunch or dinner. For an easy variation, leave out the mushrooms and cheese and add ½ cup chopped spinach or kale.

- 6 cups chicken broth
- ½ cup scallions, cut into ¼-inch-thick slices
- 4 shiitake mushrooms, stems removed, wiped clean, and cut into ¼-inch-thick slices
- 1 teaspoon wheat-free tamari
- Pinch of finely ground white pepper
- 4 tablespoons Parmesan shavings or a small piece of Parmesan rind (optional)
- ½ cup (4 ounces) egg whites

1. In a medium saucepan, bring the chicken broth to a simmer. Add 6 tablespoons of the scallions, the mushrooms, tamari, and white pepper. If using a Parmesan rind, add it here. Return to a bare simmer and cook for 3 minutes.

2. Constantly stirring with a fork to create ribbons, gradually add the egg whites in a slow stream. Cook until the whites are set, about 1 minute.

3. Remove from the heat. Ladle into bowls and garnish with the remaining 2 tablespoons scallions. Sprinkle with Parmesan shavings, if using, and serve.

Egg, Bacon, and Spinach Salad

Makes 6 Servings

You can have (some) bacon and eat it, too. Let this recipe serve as inspiration to get creative with ways to add more vegetables to your favorite proteins. Camelina oil, a newer oil on the market, is high in Omega-3 but loses its nutritional benefits when heated. Use it here to make the dressing. It is available at specialty markets.

- 2 tablespoons olive oil, plus ¼ cup olive or camelina oil
- ½ cup (4 ounces) egg whites
- ¼ pound slab bacon, cut into ¼-inch-thick slices
- 1 garlic clove, minced
- 1 small shallot, finely chopped
- Juice of ½ lemon
- 1½ tablespoons sherry vinegar
- 1 tablespoon chopped fresh flat-leaf parsley
- 1 teaspoon sea salt
- ¼ teaspoon freshly ground black pepper
- Two 5-ounce packages baby spinach

1. Warm 2 tablespoons olive oil in a sauté pan over medium-high heat. Add the egg whites and cook until set, about 3 minutes. Set aside. Cook the bacon in a heavy skillet over medium-high heat until golden brown and crisp, 6 to 8 minutes. Transfer the bacon to a plate lined with paper towels. Reserve 1 teaspoon bacon fat and discard the rest.

2. Meanwhile, combine the garlic, shallot, lemon juice, and sherry vinegar in a small bowl. Whisk in ¼ cup olive or camelina oil; add the parsley, salt, and pepper.

3. In a large bowl, toss together the spinach, cooked bacon, reserved warm bacon fat, vinaigrette, and cooked egg whites. Season with salt and pepper, if necessary, and serve immediately.

Salmon Scramble Sandwich

Makes 1 Serving

Any smoked fish or shellfish works well in this recipe. Feel free to substitute trout, sardines, herring, or oysters for the salmon.

- 1 tablespoon pistachio oil
- 1 tablespoon finely chopped red onion
- ½ cup (4 ounces) egg whites, beaten
- 1 tablespoon finely chopped dill
- ½ teaspoon capers, rinsed and chopped
- 1 ounce smoked salmon
- 1 slice tomato
- 1 slice spelt, rye, or emmer bread

1. Heat the pistachio oil in a small nonstick skillet over medium heat. Add the red onion and cook, stirring, until it begins to soften, about 1 minute. Add the egg whites, dill, and capers and cook, stirring occasionally, until whites are set, about 2 minutes.

2. To assemble the sandwich, layer the scrambled eggs, smoked salmon, and tomato on the bread.

11

CHOCOLATE

Mexican Hot Chocolate (Chocolate Caliente)

Makes 4 Servings

To benefit from chocolate's natural flavonoids, look for dark chocolate that has not undergone Dutch processing.

- 4½ cups unsweetened almond milk

- 5 ounces dark chocolate (70 percent cocoa), chopped
- ¼ teaspoon ground cinnamon

---

1. Heat the almond milk in a saucepan over medium heat to just below the simmering point. Then add the chocolate. When the chocolate has melted, add the cinnamon.

2. Whisk vigorously and serve immediately.

Dark-Chocolate Nut Clusters

Makes 32 Pieces

Combine rich macadamia nuts with sweet dark chocolate for a decadent dessert that is actually good for you. The hint of sea salt only adds to the pleasure.

- 1 cup plus 3 tablespoons melted dark chocolate (70 percent cocoa)
- 1½ cups whole macadamia nuts
- Coarse sea salt or lavender sea salt, to taste

1. Line a baking sheet with parchment paper or a baking mat. Place 1 teaspoon of the melted chocolate on the paper; top with a small handful of macadamia nuts. Drizzle the nuts with 1 tablespoon of the melted chocolate.

2. Repeat the process with the remaining macadamia nuts and chocolate. Sprinkle with the salt. Transfer to the refrigerator and chill until firm.

Chocolate Pudding

Makes 4 Servings

For a satisfying, lip-smacking dessert, nothing beats chocolate pudding. Arrowroot is a thickening agent similar to cornstarch.

- 3 teaspoons arrowroot
- 1 to 2 tablespoons lukewarm water
- ¼ cup organic sugar
- ¼ cup non-alkalized cocoa powder
- Pinch of salt
- 2 cups unsweetened almond milk
- ⅓ cup dairy-free chocolate chips
- ½ teaspoon pure vanilla extract or almond extract

1. In a small cup or bowl, combine the arrowroot with the water, mixing to dissolve. Set aside.

2. In a small saucepan, combine the sugar, cocoa powder, and salt. Over medium-low heat, gradually add the almond milk, about ¼ cup at a time, stirring constantly until smooth. Cook until a thin film develops on top of the liquid and steam rises from the surface, but do not let the mixture boil. Remove the pan from heat. Add the chocolate chips, stirring constantly until the chocolate has melted.

3. Mix in the arrowroot mixture and vanilla and return the pan to the stove over medium-low heat. Stirring constantly, cook until the mixture is thick but just slightly thinner than desired. Transfer the pudding to a heatproof dish to cool. Place plastic wrap directly on the surface to prevent a skin from forming.

Flourless Chocolate Cake

Makes 1 (9-Inch) Torta

By all accounts, torta caprese, *the best-known Italian version of flourless chocolate cake, originated by accident on the island of Capri. No one knows exactly how it happened: There are tales of bakers who mistook cocoa powder or ground almonds for flour, and of cooks simply forgetting to add flour. Whatever went down, the result is a chocoholic's dream. Gelato, ice cream, and whipped cream make great toppings.*

- 1¾ cups blanched almonds
- ¼ cup unsweetened cocoa powder
- 1 tablespoon vanilla extract
- 1 cup granulated sugar
- 5 eggs, room temperature
- 8 ounces high-quality dark chocolate (not unsweetened), chopped into small pieces
- 1 cup (2 sticks) unsalted butter
- Confectioners' sugar for dusting

1. Preheat the oven to 350°F. Line the bottom of a 9-inch regular or spring-form cake pan with a round of parchment paper or wax paper.

2. Spread the almonds in a single layer on a baking sheet, and toast on the middle rack of oven until golden, 8 to 10 minutes. Let cool in the pan; then grind in a food processor or coffee grinder and set aside. You should end up with 1¼ to 1½ cups.

3. In a large mixing bowl, combine cocoa powder, vanilla, and sugar. Beat in eggs one at a time, mixing thoroughly, and set aside.

continued ▶

Flourless Chocolate Cake *continued* ▶

4. Melt chocolate and butter in a double boiler, or in a metal or glass bowl fit snugly on top of a medium saucepan: Fill the saucepan or the bottom of the double boiler with 2 or 3 inches of water. The water should not touch the upper container. Set the lower pot over low heat, and bring the water to a low simmer; then turn off the heat, place the upper container on top, and put in the chocolate. When the chocolate starts to melt, begin stirring gently and steadily. Let almost all of the chocolate melt; then remove the upper container from its place on the stove to the counter. Continue stirring until chocolate and butter are completely melted into a satiny cream.

5. Whisk melted chocolate into the cocoa-egg mixture, and then add almonds. Pour the batter into the pan, spread it evenly, and smooth it out on top. Bake until the cake starts separating from the side of the pan and a knife inserted in the center comes out with only a few moist crumbs, about 50 minutes. Set the pan on a wire rack, and let the cake cool for 5 minutes; then invert the pan onto another rack to release the cake. Peel off the parchment or wax paper and discard. When the cake has cooled completely, invert onto a serving plate and dust with confectioners' sugar.

INDEX